ESSENTIAI HAEMATOLOGY

A. V. Hoffbrand MA DM FRCP FRCPath
Professor of Haematology, Royal Free Hospital
and School of Medicine, London

J. E. Pettit MD FRCPA FRCPath
Associate Professor of Haematology,
University of Otago, Dunedin, New Zealand

Second Edition

Blackwell Scientific Publications
Oxford London
Edinburgh Boston Melbourne

© 1980, 1984 by
Blackwell Scientific Publications
Editorial Offices:
Osney Mead, Oxford OX2 OEL
8 John Street, London WC1N 2ES
23 Ainslie Place, Edinburgh EH3 6AJ
3 Cambridge Center, Suite 208
    Cambridge, Massachusetts 02142, USA
107 Barry Street, Carlton
    Victoria 3053, Australia

First published 1980
Reprinted 1981, 1982, 1983 (twice)
Second edition 1984
Reprinted 1985
Reprinted with corrections 1985,
    1988 (twice) and 1989
German edition 1986
Japanese edition 1987

Printed and bound
in Great Britain by
William Clowes Limited
Beccles and London

DISTRIBUTORS

Marston Book Services Ltd
PO Box 87
Oxford OX2 0DT

USA
Year Book Medical Publishers
200 North LaSalle Street
Chicago, Illinois 60601

Canada
The C. V. Mosby Company
5240 Finch Avenue East
Scarborough, Ontario

Australia
Blackwell Scientific Publications
(Australia) Pty Ltd
107 Barry Street
Carlton, Victoria 3053

British Library
Cataloguing in Publication Data

Hoffbrand, A.V.
    Essential Haematology.—2nd ed.
    1. Haematology
    I. Title   II. Pettit, J.E.
    616.1 5   R145

ISBN 0–632–01196–3

Contents

Preface to first edition

The major changes that have occurred in all fields of medicine over the last decade have been accompanied by an increased understanding of the biochemical, physiological and immunological processes involved in normal blood cell formation and function and the disturbances that may occur in different diseases. At the same time, the range of treatment available for patients with diseases of the blood and blood forming organs has widened and improved substantially as understanding of the disease processes has increased and new drugs and means of support care have been introduced.

We hope the present book will enable the medical student of the 1980s to grasp the essential features of modern clinical and laboratory haematology and to achieve an understanding of how many of the manifestations of blood diseases can be explained with this new knowledge of the disease processes.

We would like to thank many colleagues and assistants who have helped with the preparation of the book. In particular, Dr H. G. Prentice cared for the patients whose haematological responses are illustrated in Figures 5.3 and 7.8 and Dr J. McLaughlin supplied Figure 8.6. Dr S. Knowles reviewed critically the final manuscript and made many helpful suggestions. Any remaining errors are, however, our own. We also thank Mr J. B. Irwin and R. W. McPhee who drew many excellent diagrams, Mr Cedric Gilson for expert photomicrography, Mrs T. Charalambos, Mrs B. Elliot, Mrs M. Evans and Miss J. Allaway for typing the manuscript, and Mr Jony Russell of Blackwell Scientific Publications for his invaluable help and patience.

A. V. Hoffbrand
J. E. Pettit

vii

Preface to second edition

Although it is only four years since the appearance of the first edition of this short textbook for medical students, a number of major advances have been made in the understanding of fundamental mechanisms in blood cell formation and function, and of the aetiology and treatment of blood disorders. In order to incorporate this new information, it was felt necessary to rewrite the text in all sections with major changes to the chapters on haemoglobinopathies, white cells, leukaemia, lymphoma and haemostasis. There are 52 new or revised figures and new tables have been incorporated throughout. Nevertheless, we hope the book has maintained its original objectives by omitting all non-essential detail.

We wish to thank in particular Professor G. Janossy, Drs Marcella Contrerras, R. Dick, J. M. Faed, P. B. A. Kernoff, E. G. D. Tuddenham for advice on revisions in various sections of the manuscript and Miss J. Allaway, Mrs M. Evans and Mrs B. Elliot for typing the new manuscript. We are also grateful to the publishers, particularly Peter Saugman and Jony Russell for their enthusiastic support and help.

A. V. H.
J. E. P.

Normal values

	Units	Males	Females
Haemoglobin	g/dl	13.5–17.5	11.5–15.5
Red cells (erythrocytes)	× 10^{12}/l	4.5–6.5	3.9–5.6
PCV (haematocrit)	%	40–52	36–48
MCV	fl	80–95	
MCH	pg	27–34	
MCHC	g/dl	30–35	
White cells (leucocytes)—total	× 10^9/l	4.0–11.0	
neutrophils		2.5–7.5	
lymphocytes		1.5–3.5	
monocytes		0.2–0.8	
eosinophils		0.04–0.44	
basophils		0.01–0.1	
Platelets	× 10^9/l	150–400	
Red cell mass		30 ± 5 ml/kg	25 ± 5 ml/kg
Plasma volume		45 ± 5 ml/kg	45 ± 5 ml/kg
Serum iron		10–30 μmol/l	
Total iron binding capacity		40–75 μmol/l	(2.0–4.0 g/l as transferrin)
Serum ferritin	μg/l	40–340	14–150
Serum vitamin B$_{12}$	ng/l	160–925	
Serum folate	μg/l	3.0–15.0	
Red cell folate	μg/l	160–640	

Chapter 1
Blood cell formation (haemopoiesis)

This first chapter mainly concerns the production and metabolism of red cells (erythrocytes) and general aspects of anaemia. However, as red cells are formed after many cell divisions from the same stem cells that give rise to all blood cells, it is important to consider first some general aspects of blood cell formation (haemopoiesis).

Site

In the first few weeks of gestation the yolk-sac is the main site of haemopoiesis. From six weeks until 6–7 months of foetal life the liver and spleen are the main organs involved and they continue to produce blood cells until about two weeks after birth (Table 1.1). The bone marrow is the most important site from 6–7 months of foetal life and, during normal childhood and adult

Table 1.1 Sites of haemopoiesis.

Foetus	0–2 months—yolk sac
	2–7 months—liver, spleen
	5–9 months—bone marrow
Infants	Bone marrow (practically all bones)
Adults	Vertebrae, ribs, sternum, skull, sacrum and pelvis, proximal ends of femur

life, the marrow is the only source of new blood cells. The developing cells are situated outside the bone marrow sinuses and mature cells are released into the sinus spaces, the marrow microcirculation and so into the general circulation.

In infancy, all the bone marrow is haemopoietic but, during childhood, there is progressive fatty replacement of marrow throughout the long bones so that, in adult life, haemopoietic marrow is confined to the central skeleton (Table 1.1). Even in these haemopoietic areas, approximately 50% of the marrow consists of fat (Fig. 1.1). The remaining fatty marrow is capable of reversion to haemopoiesis and in many diseases there is also

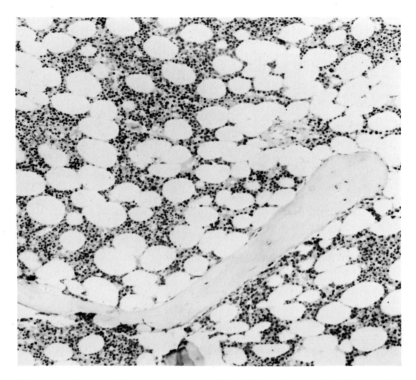

Fig. 1.1 A normal bone marrow trephine biopsy (posterior iliac crest). Haematoxylin and eosin stain; approximately 50% of the intertrabecular tissue is haemopoietic tissue and 50% is fat.

expansion of haemopoiesis down the long bones. Moreover, the liver and spleen can resume their foetal haemopoietic role (so-called 'extramedullary haemopoiesis').

Haemopoietic stem cells

It is now thought that a common (pluripotential) stem cell gives rise after a number of cell divisions and differentiation steps to a series of progenitor cells for three main marrow cell lines: **a** erythroid; **b** granulocytic and monocytic; and **c** megakarocytic, as well as to a common lymphoid stem cell (Fig. 1.2). Although the appearance of the pluripotential stem cells is probably similar to that of small or intermediate-sized lymphocytes, their presence can be shown by culture techniques. The existence of the separate progenitor cells for the three cell lines has also been demonstrated by in-vitro culture techniques. The earliest detectable myeloid precursor gives rise to granulocytes, erythroblasts, monocytes and megakaryocytes and is termed CFU_{GEMM} (CFU = colony forming unit in culture medium, Fig. 1.2). More mature and specialised

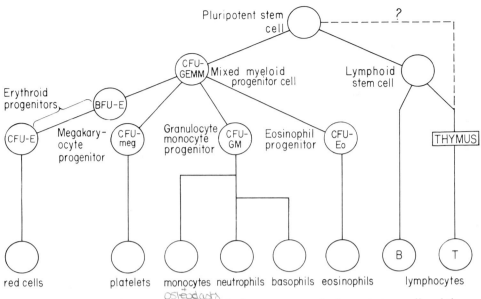

Fig. 1.2 Diagrammatic representation of the bone marrow pluripotent stem cell and the cell lines that arise from it. Various progenitor cells can now be identified by culture in semi-solid medium by the type of colony they form.
C F U = colony forming unit, G E M M = mixed granulocyte, erythroid, monocyte, megakaryocyte, E = erythroid, meg = megakaryocyte, G M = granulocyte/monocyte, Eo = eosinophil, B F U–E = burst forming unit, erythroid.

progenitors are termed CFU_{GM} (granulocytes and monocytes), CFU_{Eo} (eosinophils). CFU_e (erythroid) and CFU_{meg} (megakaryocyte). BFU_e (burst forming unit, erythroid) refers to an earlier erythroid progenitor than the CFU_e (see Fig. 1.2). The stem cell also has the capability of self-renewal so that, although the marrow is a major site of new cell production, its overall cellularity remains constant in a normal healthy steady state. The precursor cells are, however, capable of responding to various stimuli and hormonal messages with increased production of one or other cell line when the need arises.

The bone marrow is a suitable environment for stem cell growth and development. This is provided for by stromal cells, fat cells and a microvascular network. If, for instance, haemopoietic stem cells are infused intravenously into a suitably prepared recipient, they seed the marrow successfully but do not thrive at other sites. This is the basis of bone marrow transplantation now carried out for a number of serious bone marrow diseases.

The bone marrow is also the primary site of origin of lymphocytes in humans (Chapter 6) and there is evidence for a common precursor cell of both the haemopoietic and lymphoid systems. Haemopoietic stem cells also give rise to osteoclasts which are part of the the monocyte phagocyte system. The development of the mature cells, the granulocytes, monocytes, megakaryocytes and lymphocytes, is further considered in other sections of this book. Erythropoiesis is dealt with next.

ERYTHROPOIESIS

The earliest recognisable erythroid cell in the marrow is the pronormoblast which—on the usual Romanowsky (e.g. May–Grünwald Giemsa, Leishman or Wright) stain—is a large cell with dark-blue cytoplasm, a central nucleus with nucleoli and slightly clumped chromatin. By a number of cell divisions, this gives rise to a series of progressively smaller normoblasts. They also contain progressively more haemoglobin (which stains pink) in the cytoplasm; the cytoplasm stains paler blue as it loses its RNA and protein synthetic apparatus while the nuclear chromatin becomes more condensed (Fig. 1.3a & b). The nucleus is finally extruded from the late normoblast within the marrow and a reticulocyte stage results which still contains some ribosomal RNA and is still able to synthesise haemoglobin (Figs. 1.4 & 1.5). This cell spends 1–2 days in the marrow and also circulates in the peripheral blood for 1–2 days before maturing, mainly in the spleen, when RNA is completely lost and a completely pink-staining, mature erythrocyte (red

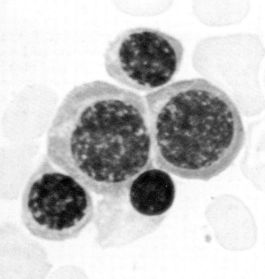

Fig. 1.3a Photomicrograph of normal bone marrow red cell precursors (normoblasts).

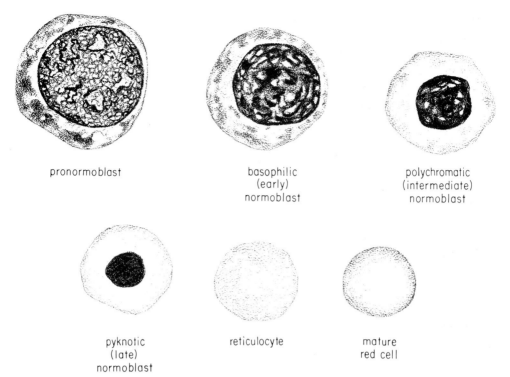

pronormoblast

basophilic
(early)
normoblast

polychromatic
(intermediate)
normoblast

pyknotic
(late)
normoblast

reticulocyte

mature
red cell

Fig. 1.3b The red cell series (diagrammatic). There is progressive condensation of the nucleus which is extruded at the late normoblast stage. The cytoplasm contains progressively less RNA and more haemoglobin.

cell) results which is a non-nucleated biconcave disc. A single pronormoblast usually gives rise to 16 mature red cells (Fig. 1.4). Nucleated red cells (normoblasts) appear in the blood if erythropoiesis is occurring outside the marrow (extramedullary erythropoiesis) and also with some marrow diseases. Normoblasts are not present in normal human peripheral blood.

Erythropoietin

Erythropoietic activity is regulated by the hormone erythropoietin, which is produced by the combination of a renal factor with a plasma protein. The stimulus to erythropoietin production is the O_2 tension in the tissues of the kidney. When anaemia occurs, or haemoglobin for some metabolic reason is unable to give up O_2 normally, erythropoietin production increases and stimulates erythropoiesis by:

1 Increasing the number of stem cells committed to erythropoiesis. The proportion of erythroid cells in the marrow increases and, in the chronic state, there is anatomical expansion of eryth-

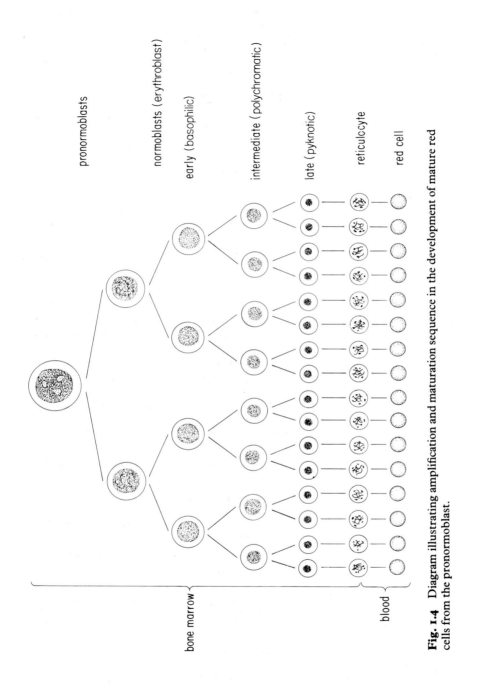

Fig. 1.4 Diagram illustrating amplification and maturation sequence in the development of mature red cells from the pronormoblast.

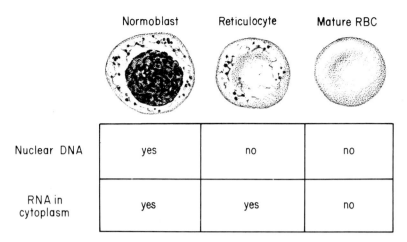

	Normoblast	Reticulocyte	Mature RBC
Nuclear DNA	yes	no	no
RNA in cytoplasm	yes	yes	no

Fig. 1.5 Comparison of the DNA and RNA content of the erythroblast (normoblast), reticulocyte and mature red cell (erythrocyte, RBC).

roid tissue down the long bones and sometimes into extramedullary sites. In infants, the marrow cavity may expand into cortical bone and bone deformities result, e.g. frontal bossing and protrusion of the maxilla (see p. 76).

2 Increasing haemoglobin synthesis in red cell precursors.

3 Decreasing maturation time of red cell precursors.

4 Releasing marrow reticulocytes into peripheral blood at an earlier stage than normal ('shift reticulocytes').

On the other hand, increased O_2 supply to the tissues due to an increased red cell mass or because haemoglobin is able to release its O_2 more readily than normal reduces the erythropoietin drive.

Substances needed for erythropoiesis

Because of the very great numbers of new red cells that are produced each day, the marrow requires many precursors to synthesise the new cells and the large amounts of haemoglobin. The following groups of substances are needed:

1 *Metals:* Iron, manganese, cobalt.

2 *Vitamins:* Vitamin B_{12} (B_{12}), folate, vitamin C, vitamin E, vitamin B_6 (pyridoxine), thiamine, riboflavin, pantothenic acid.

3 *Amino acids.*

4 *Hormones:* erythropoietin, androgens, thyroxine.

Well recognised anaemias occur with iron, B_{12} or folate deficiencies. Anaemias also occur with amino acid (protein), thyroxine or androgen deficiency but these may be adaptations to the lower tissue O_2 consumption, rather than a direct effect of the deficiency on erythropoiesis. Anaemia also occurs in the deficiency of vitamin C (scurvy), vitamin E and riboflavin, but it is not clear whether these are purely due to an effect of these deficiences on erythropoiesis. B_6 responsive anaemias also occur (see p. 40) but these are not usually due to B_6 deficiency.

Haemoglobin synthesis

The main function of red cells is to carry O_2 to the tissues and to return carbon dioxide (CO_2) from the tissues to the lungs. In order to achieve this gaseous exchange, they contain a specialised protein, haemoglobin. Each red cell contains approximately 640 million haemoglobin molecules and each molecule of normal adult haemoglobin (Hb A) consists of four polypeptide chains $\alpha_2\beta_2$, each with its own haem group. The mol. wt. of Hb A is 68 000. Normal adult blood also contains small quantities of two other haemoglobins, Hb F and Hb A_2 which also contain α chains but γ and δ chains respectively instead of β (Table 1.2). In the embryo and

Table 1.2 Normal haemoglobins in adult blood.

	A	F	A_2
Structure	$\alpha_2\beta_2$	$\alpha_2\gamma_2$	$\alpha_2\delta_2$
Normal (%)	96–98	0.5–0.8	1.5–3.2

foetus, haemoglobins Gower 1, Gower 2, Portland and foetal dominate at different stages. The genes for these globin chains occur in two clusters, the β, δ, γ, ε cluster on chromosome 11 and the α, ζ cluster on chromosome 16 (Fig. 1.6). The major switch from foetal to adult haemoglobin occurs 3–6 months after birth. Sixty-five per cent of haemoglobin is synthesised in the erythroblasts and 35% at the reticulocyte stage.

Haem synthesis occurs largely in the mitochondria by a series of biochemical reactions commencing with the condensation of glycine and succinyl coenzyme A under the action of the key rate-limiting enzyme delta-amino laevulinic acid (ALA)-synthetase (Fig. 1.7). Pyridoxal phosphate (vitamin B_6) is a coenzyme for this reaction which is stimulated by erythropoietin and inhibited by haem. Ultimately, protoporphyrin combines with iron to form haem (Fig. 1.8) each molecule of which combines with a globin chain made on the polyribosomes (Fig. 1.7). A tetramer of four globin chains each with its own haem group in a 'pocket' is then formed to make up a haemoglobin molecule (Fig. 1.9).

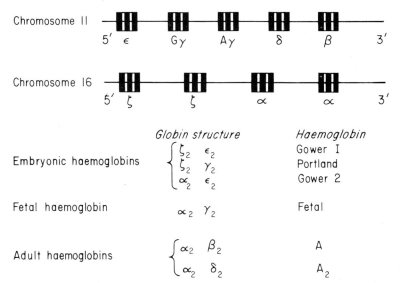

Fig. 1.6 Diagrammatic representation of the globin gene arrangements on chromosomes 11 and 16.

5′, 3′ refer to the direction of the deoxyribose sugar binding. The ζ, α, β, γ, δ and ε genes have been shown to have coding sequences, 'extrons', shown in solid bars and intervening, non-coding sequences, 'introns', shown in open bars. The combinations of these genes coding for the various haemoglobin tetramer molecules found in embryonic, foetal and adult life are also shown. Gγ and Aγ refers to the two types of foetal globin chain with either glycine or alanine at position 136.

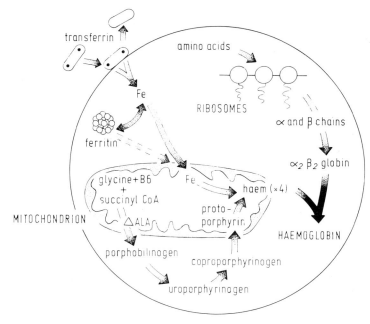

Fig. 1.7 Haemoglobin synthesis in the developing red cell. The mitochondria are the main site of protoporphyrin synthesis, iron is supplied from circulating transferrin and globin chains are synthesised on ribosomes. △ALA = delta-amino laevulinic acid.

Blood cell formation (haemopoiesis)   9

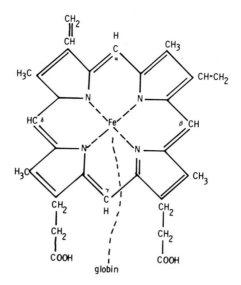

Fig. 1.8 The structure of haem.

Haemoglobin function

The red cells in systemic arterial blood carry oxygen from the lungs to the tissues and return in venous blood with carbon dioxide (CO_2) to the lungs. As the haemoglobin molecule loads and unloads O_2, the individual globin chains in the haemoglobin molecule move on each other (Fig. 1.9). When O_2 is unloaded, the β chains are pulled apart, permitting entry of the metabolite 2,3 diphosphoglycerate (2,3-DPG) resulting in a lower affinity of the molecule

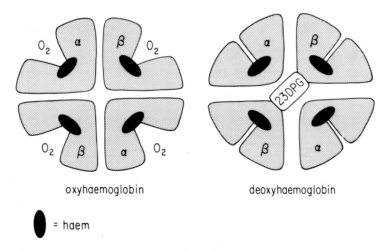

oxyhaemoglobin   deoxyhaemoglobin

● = haem

Fig. 1.9 The oxygenated and deoxygenated haemoglobin molecule.
2,3 DPG = 2,3 diphosphoglycerate
α,β = globin chains of normal adult haemoglobin (Hb A).

for O_2. This movement is responsible for the sigmoid form of the haemoglobin O_2-dissociation curve (Fig. 1.10). The P_{50} (i.e. the partial pressure of O_2 at which the haemoglobin is half saturated with O_2) of normal blood is 26.6 mmHg. With increased affinity for O_2, the curve shifts to the left (i.e. the P_{50} falls) while, with decreased affinity for O_2, the curve shifts to the right (i.e. the P_{50} rises).

Normally *in vivo*, O_2 exchange operates between 95% saturation (arterial blood) with a mean arterial O_2 tension of 95 mmHg and

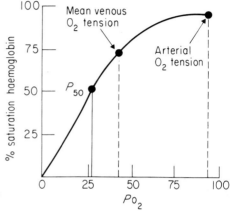

Fig. 1.10 The haemoglobin oxygen-dissociation curve.

70% saturation (venous blood) with a mean venous O_2 tension of 40 mmHg.

The normal position of the curve depends on the concentration of 2,3-DPG, H^+ ions and CO_2 in the red cell and on the structure of the haemoglobin molecule. High concentrations of 2,3-DPG, H^+ or CO_2, and the presence of certain haemoglobins, e.g. sickle haemoglobin (Hb S) shift the curve to the right whereas foetal haemoglobin (Hb F)—which is unable to bind 2,3-DPG—and certain rare abnormal haemoglobins associated with polycyth-aemia shift the curve to the left because they give up O_2 less readily than normal.

THE RED CELL

In order successfully to carry haemoglobin into close contact with the tissues and for successful gaseous exchange, the red cell, 8 μm in diameter, must be able to pass repeatedly through the micro-circulation whose minimum diameter is 3.5 μm, to maintain haemoglobin in a reduced state and to maintain osmotic equilib-rium despite the high concentration of protein (haemoglobin) in the cell. Its total journey throughout its 120 day lifespan has been

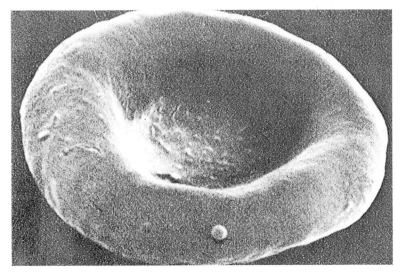

Fig. 1.11 A scanning electronmicroscopic view of a normal red cell.

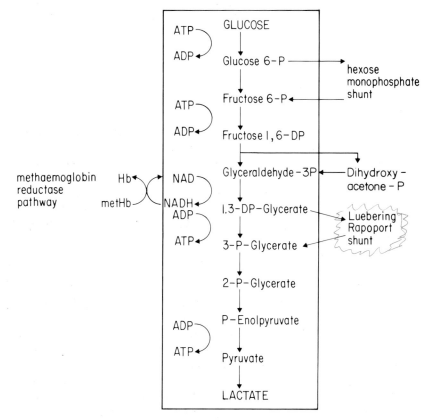

Fig. 1.12 The Embden–Meyerhof glycolytic pathway.

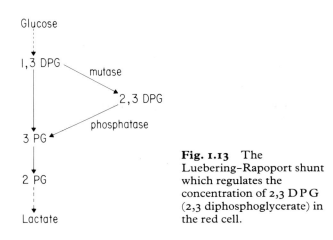

Glucose

1,3 DPG — mutase

2,3 DPG

phosphatase

3 PG

2 PG

Lactate

Fig. 1.13 The Luebering–Rapoport shunt which regulates the concentration of 2,3 DPG (2,3 diphosphoglycerate) in the red cell.

estimated to be 300 miles. To fulfill these functions, the cell is a flexible, biconcave disc (Fig. 1.11) with an ability to generate energy as ATP by the anaerobic, glycolytic (Embden–Meyerhof) pathway (Fig. 1.12) and to generate reducing power as NADH by this pathway and as NADPH by the hexose monophosphate shunt (Fig. 1.14).

Red cell metabolism

EMBDEN–MEYERHOF PATHWAY

In this series of biochemical reactions glucose is metabolised to lactate (Fig. 1.12). For each molecule of glucose used, two molecules of ATP and thus two high-energy phosphate bonds are generated. This ATP provides energy for maintenance of red cell volume, shape and flexibility. The red cell has an osmotic pressure five times that of plasma and an inherent weakness of the membrane results in continual Na^+ and K^+ movement. A membrane ATPase sodium pump is needed, and this uses one molecule of ATP to move three sodium ions out and two potassium ions into the cell.

The Embden–Meyerhof pathway also generates NADH which is needed by the enzyme methaemoglobin reductase to reduce functionally dead methaemoglobin (oxidized haemoglobin) containing ferric ($Fe^{III}OH$) iron (produced by oxidation of about 3% of haemoglobin each day) to functionally active, reduced haemoglobin (containing ferrous, Fe^{II}, iron). 2,3-DPG which is generated in the shunt, or side-arm, of this pathway (Fig. 1.13) forms a 1:1 complex with haemoglobin and, as mentioned earlier, is important in the regulation of haemoglobin's oxygen affinity.

About 5% of glycolysis occurs by this oxidative pathway in which glucose 6-phosphate is converted to 6-phosphogluconate and so to ribulose 5-phosphate (Fig. 1.14). NADPH is generated and is linked with glutathione which maintains sulphydril ($-SH$) groups intact in the cell including those in haemoglobin and the

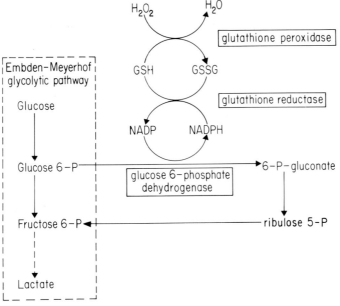

Fig. 1.14 The hexose monophosphate shunt pathway.

red cell membrane. NADPH is also used by another methaemoglobin reductase to maintain haemoglobin iron in the functionally active Fe^{++} state. In one of the commonest inherited abnormalities of red cells, glucose 6-phosphate dehydrogenase (G6PD) deficiency, the red cells are extremely susceptible to oxidant stress (see p. 66).

Red cell membrane

This is a bipolar lipid layer containing structural and contractile proteins and numerous enzymes and surface antigens (Fig. 1.15). About 50% of the membrane is protein, 40% is fats and up to 10% is carbohydrate. The lipids consist of 60% phospholipid, 30% neutral lipids (mainly cholesterol) and 10% glycolipids. The phospho- and glycolipids are structural with polar groups on the external and internal surfaces and non-polar groups at the centre of the membrane. Carbohydrates occur only on the external surface while proteins are thought to be either peripheral or to be

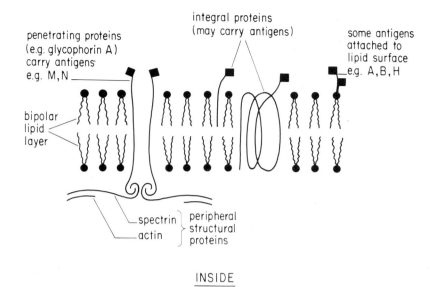

penetrating proteins
(e.g. glycophorin A)
carry antigens
e.g. M,N

integral proteins
(may carry antigens)

some antigens
attached to
lipid surface
e.g. A,B,H

bipolar
lipid
layer

spectrin
actin

peripheral
structural
proteins

INSIDE

Fig. 1.15 A simplified diagram of the protein and lipid structure of the red cell membrane.

integral, penetrating the lipid bilayer. One of the proteins — spectrin — is thought to be structural on the inner surface, maintaining the biconcave shape. Defects of this protein may explain some of the abnormalities of shape of the red cell membrane, e.g. hereditary spherocytosis and elliptocytosis (see Chapter 4), while alterations in lipid composition due to congenital or acquired abnormalities in plasma cholesterol or phospholipid may be associated with other membrane abnormalities. For instance, an increase in cholesterol and phospholipid has been suggested as one cause of target cells whereas a large selective increase in cholesterol may cause acanthocyte formation (*see* Fig. 1.17a).

Red cell destruction

This occurs after a mean lifespan of 120 days when the cells are removed extravascularly by the macrophages of the reticulo-endothelial (RE) system, especially in the marrow but also in the liver and spleen. Red cell metabolism gradually deteriorates as enzymes are not replaced, until the cells become non-viable, but the exact reason why the red cells die is obscure. The breakdown of red cells liberates iron for recirculation via plasma transferrin to marrow erythroblasts, and protoporphyrin which is broken down to bilirubin. This circulates to the liver where it is conjugated to glucuronides which are excreted into the gut via bile and converted to stercobilinogen and stercobilin (excreted in faeces) (Fig. 1.16). Stercobilinogen and stercobilin are partly re-absorbed and excreted in urine as urobilinogen and urobilin. A small fraction

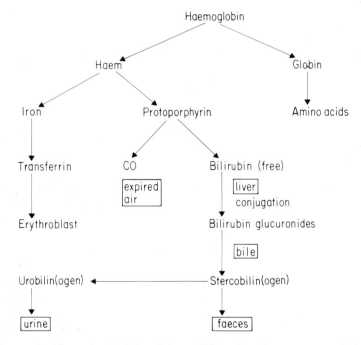

Fig. 1.16 Normal red cell breakdown. This takes place extravascularly in the macrophages of the reticulo-endothelial (RE) system.

of protoporphyrin is converted to carbon monoxide (CO) and excreted via the lungs. Globin chains are broken down to amino acids which are reutilised for general protein synthesis in the body. Intravascular haemolysis (breakdown of red cells within blood vessels) plays little or no part in normal red cell destruction.

ANAEMIA

This is normally defined as a haemoglobin concentration in blood of less than 13.5 g/dl in adult males and less than 11.5 g/dl in adult females, although some use 14.0 g/dl and 12.0 g/dl as the adult lower limits of normal. From the age of 3 months to puberty, less than 11.0 g/dl indicates anaemia. As newborn infants have a high haemoglobin level, 15.0 g/dl is taken as the lower limit at birth (Table 1.3). Reduction of haemoglobin is usually accompanied by a fall in red cell count and packed cell volume (PCV) but these

Table 1.3 Normal adult red cell values.

	Male	Female
Haemoglobin (Hb)* (g/dl)	13.5-17.5	11.5-15.5
Haematocrit (PCV) (%)	40-52	36-48
Red cell count (× 10^{12}/l)	4.5-6.5	3.9-5.6
Mean cell haemoglobin (MCH) (pg)	27-34	
Mean cell volume (MCV) (fl)	80-95	
Mean cell haemoglobin concentration (MCHC) (g/dl)	30-35	

Children: Newborn   Hb 15.0-21.0 g/dl
  3 months   Hb 9.5-12.5 g/dl
  1 year-puberty   Hb 11.0-13.5 g/dl

may be normal in some patients with subnormal haemoglobin levels (and therefore by definition anaemic). Alterations in total circulating plasma volume as well as of total circulating haemoglobin mass determine whether or not anaemia is present. Reduction in plasma volume (as in dehydration) may mask anaemia; conversely, an increase in plasma volume (as with splenomegaly) may cause anaemia even with a normal total circulating red cell and haemoglobin mass.

After acute major blood loss, anaemia is not immediately apparent since the total blood volume is reduced. It takes up to a day for the plasma volume to be replaced and so for the degree of anaemia to become apparent. Regeneration of the haemoglobin mass takes substantially longer. The initial clinical features of major blood loss are, therefore, due to reduction in blood volume rather than to anaemia.

Clinical features

In some patients with quite severe anaemia there may be no symptoms or signs whereas others with mild anaemia may be severely incapacitated. The presence or absence of clinical features can be considered under four major headings: (i) the speed of onset of anaemia, (ii) the severity of anaemia, (iii) the age of the patient, and (iv) the haemoglobin oxygen-dissociation curve.

(i) Rapidly progressive anaemia causes more symptoms than anaemia of slow onset because there is less time for adaptation in the cardiovascular system and in the oxygen-dissociation curve of the haemoglobin.
(ii) Mild anaemia often produces no symptoms or signs but these are usually present when the haemoglobin is less than 9–10 g/dl. Even severe anaemia (haemoglobin concentration as low as 6.0 g/dl) may produce remarkably few symptoms, however, when there is very gradual onset in a young subject who is otherwise healthy.
(iii) The elderly tolerate anaemia less well than the young because

of the effect of lack of oxygen on organs when normal cardiovascular compensation (increased cardiac output due to increased stroke volume and tachycardia) is impaired.

(iv) Anaemia, in general, is associated with a rise in 2,3-DPG in the red cells and a shift in the O_2-dissociation curve to the right so that oxygen is given up more readily to tissues. This adaptation is particularly marked in some anaemias which either affect red cell metabolism directly, e.g. in the anaemia of pyruvate kinase deficiency (which causes a rise in 2,3-DPG concentration in the red cells) or which are associated with a low affinity haemoglobin (e.g. haemoglobin S).

SYMPTOMS. If the patient does have symptoms, these are usually shortness of breath (particularly on exercise), weakness, lethargy, palpitation and headaches. In older subjects symptoms of cardiac failure, angina pectoris or intermittent claudication or confusion may be present. Visual disturbances due to retinal haemorrhages may complicate very severe anaemia, particularly of rapid onset.

SIGNS. These may be divided into general and specific. General signs include pallor of mucous membranes which occurs if the haemoglobin level is less than 9–10 g/dl. Skin colour, on the other hand, is not a reliable sign of anaemia, the state of the skin circulation rather than the haemoglobin content of the blood, largely determining skin colour. A hyperdynamic circulation may be present with tachycardia, a bounding pulse, cardiomegaly and a systolic flow murmur especially at the apex. Particularly in the elderly, features of congestive heart failure may be present. Retinal haemorrhages are unusual. Specific signs are associated with particular types of anaemia, e.g. koilonychia (spoon nails) with iron deficiency, jaundice with haemolytic or megaloblastic anaemias, leg ulcers with sickle cell and other haemolytic anaemias, bone deformities with thalassaemia major and other severe congenital haemolytic anaemias.

Classification and laboratory investigation

RED CELL INDICES

Although classification of anaemia based on the cause of the anaemia, e.g. failure of red cell production or excess loss or destruction of red cells, has been used, the most useful classification now that modern electronic equipment measures accurately a number of parameters of red cell size and haemoglobin content is that based on red cell indices (Table 1.4). This classification has two major advantages:

1 The type of anaemia (size of the red cells and their haemoglobin content) suggests the nature of the underlying defect and

Table 1.4 Classification of anaemia.

Microcytic, hypochromic	MCV, MCH reduced (MCV < 80 fl) (MCH < 27 pg) e.g. iron deficiency, thalassaemia (see Chapters 2 & 4).
Normocytic, normochromic	MCV, MCH normal (MCV 80–95 fl) (MCH 27–34 pg) e.g. after acute blood loss, many haemolytic anaemias and secondary anaemias, bone marrow failure (see Chapters 2 & 4). C Renal Failure!
Macrocytic	MCV raised (> 95 fl) e.g. megaloblastic anaemias (see Chapter 3).

therefore the particular investigations which would be most useful in confirming one or other diagnosis.

2 Abnormal red cell indices may suggest an underlying abnormality before anaemia as defined earlier has developed, e.g. macrocytosis (large red cells) with early vitamin B_{12} or folate deficiency. Abnormal indices may also point to an important disorder in which anaemia may not occur, e.g. some cases of thalassaemia trait in which the red cells are very small (microcytic) but because of their increased numbers the haemoglobin concentration in blood is normal.

In two common physiological situations, the mean corpuscular volume (MCV) may be outside the normal adult range. In the newborn for a few weeks the MCV is high but, in infancy, it is low (e.g. 70 fl at one year of age) and rises slowly throughout childhood to the normal adult range. In normal pregnancy there is a slight rise in MCV, even in the absence of other causes of macrocytosis, e.g. folate deficiency.

OTHER IMPORTANT INITIAL LABORATORY INVESTIGATIONS OF ANAEMIA

Although the red cell indices will point to the type of anaemia, further useful information can be obtained from the initial blood sample.

LEUCOCYTE AND PLATELET COUNTS. Measurement of these helps to distinguish 'pure' anaemia from 'pancytopenia' (a drop in red cells, granulocytes and platelets) which suggests a more general marrow defect, e.g. due to marrow hypoplasia, infiltration or general destruction of cells (e.g. hypersplenism). In anaemias due to haemolysis or haemorrhage the neutrophil and platelet counts are often raised; in infections and leukaemias the leucocyte count is also often raised and there may be abnormal leucocytes present.

RETICULOCYTE COUNT (NORMAL 0.5–2.0%; absolute count 25–75 × 10⁹/l). This should rise in anaemia and be higher the more severe the anaemia. This is particularly so when there has been time for erythroid hyperplasia to develop as in chronic haemolysis. After an acute major haemorrhage, there is an erythropoietic response in 6 hours, the reticulocyte count rises within 2–3 days, reaches a maximum in 6–10 days and remains raised until the haemoglobin returns to the normal level—providing iron deficiency or some other additional cause for anaemia is not present. If the reticulocyte count is not raised in an anaemic patient this suggests impaired marrow function or lack of erythropoietin stimulus (Table 1.5).

Table 1.5 Factors impairing the normal reticulocyte response to anaemia.

1 Marrow diseases, e.g. hypoplasia, infiltration
2 Deficiency of a haematinic, e.g. of iron, vitamin B_{12}, folate
3 Lack of erythropoietin, e.g. renal disease
4 Reduced tissue O_2 consumption, e.g. myxoedema, protein deficiency
5 Ineffective erythropoiesis, e.g. thalassaemia major, megaloblastic anaemia
6 Chronic inflammatory or malignant disease

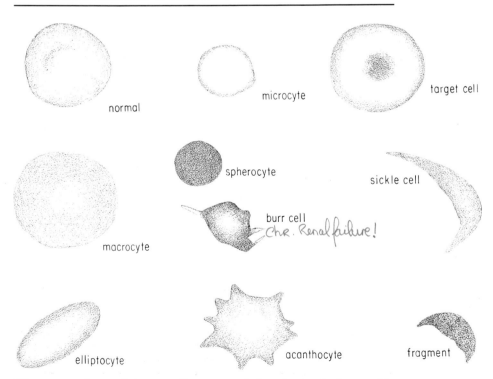

normal
microcyte
target cell
spherocyte
sickle cell
burr cell
Chr. Renal failure!
macrocyte
elliptocyte
acanthocyte
fragment

Fig. 1.17a Some of the more frequent variations in size (anisocytosis), and shape (poikilocytosis) that may be found in different anaemias.

BLOOD FILM. It is essential to examine the blood film in all cases of anaemia. Abnormal red cell morphology (Fig. 1.17a) or red cell inclusions (Fig. 1.17b) may suggest a particular diagnosis. When causes of both microcytosis and macrocytosis are present, e.g. mixed iron and folate or B_{12} deficiency, the indices may be normal but the blood film reveals a 'dimorphic' appearance (a dual population of large, well haemoglobinised cells and small, hypochromic cells). During the blood film examination the white cell differential count is performed, platelet number and morphology is assessed

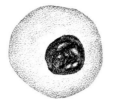

normoblast (nucleated RBC)

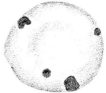
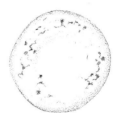

Heinz bodies
eg G6PD def
(Haemolytic A)
oxidised denatured Hb

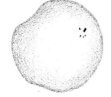

siderotic granules
contain iron

Howell–Jolly body
DNA. Remnant

reticulocyte (RNA)

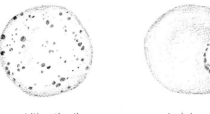

basophilic stippling
Denatured RNA.

malarial parasite

Fig. 1.17b Red cell inclusions which may be seen in the peripheral blood film in various conditions. The reticulocyte RNA and Heinz bodies are only demonstrated by supravital staining, e.g. with new methylene blue. Heinz bodies are oxidised denatured haemoglobin. Siderotic granules (Pappenheimer bodies) contain iron. The Howell–Jolly body is a DNA remnant. Basophilic stippling is denatured RNA.

Blood cell formation (haemopoiesis) 21

and the presence or absence of abnormal cells, e.g. normoblasts, granulocyte precursors, plasma cells, is noted.

BONE MARROW EXAMINATION. This may be performed by aspiration or trephine (Fig. 1.18).

Aspiration provides a film on which the detail of the developing cells can be examined (e.g. normoblastic or megaloblastic), the proportion of the different cell lines assessed (myeloid : erythroid ratio) and the presence of cells foreign to the marrow (e.g. secondary carcinoma) observed. The cellularity of the marrow can also be viewed, provided fragments are obtained. The marrow films are stained by the usual Romanowsky technique and a stain for iron is performed routinely so that the amount of iron in reticulo-endothelial stores (macrophages) and which exists as fine granules ('siderotic' granules) in the developing eythroblasts can be assessed.

Bone marrow aspiration is not required in some cases of anaemia, e.g. obvious cases of iron deficiency anaemia where more simple ancillary tests can confirm the diagnosis suspected on the peripheral blood count. But in many other cases of anaemia, as

Table 1.6 Comparison of bone marrow aspiration and trephine biopsy.

	Aspiration	Trephine
Site	Sternum Posterior iliac crest (tibia in infants)	Posterior iliac crest
Stains	Romanowsky, Perls' reaction (for iron)	Haematoxylin + Eosin Reticulin
Result Available	1–2 hours	1–7 days (according to decalcification method)
Main Indications	Investigation of anaemia, pancytopenia, suspected leukaemia, myeloma, neutropenia, thrombocytopenia, polycythaemia, etc.	Indications for additional trephine : suspicion of myelosclerosis and other myeloproliferative disorders, aplastic anaemia, malignant lymphoma, secondary carcinoma, cases of splenomegaly or pyrexia of undetermined cause. Any case where aspiration gives a 'dry' tap.
Special tests	Cytogenetics, microbiological culture, biochemical analysis, immunological and cytochemical markers.	

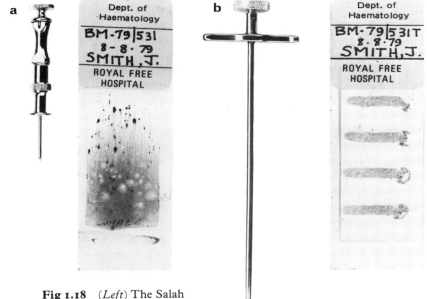

Fig 1.18 (*Left*) The Salah bone marrow aspiration needle and a smear made from a bone marrow aspirate. (*Right*) The Jamshidi bone marrow trephine needle and normal trephine sections.

well as in many other blood and systemic diseases, bone marrow aspiration often provides invaluable diagnostic help. In some conditions, the cells obtained may be used for more detailed special tests (Table 1.6).

Trephine. This provides a core of bone including marrow and is examined as a histological specimen after fixation in formalin, decalcification and sectioning. With the introduction of simple, reliable needles (e.g. Jamshidi), trephine biopsy is being used increasingly. It is less valuable than aspiration when individual cell detail is to be examined (e.g. diagnosis of megaloblastic anaemia or acute leukaemia) but provides a panoramic view of the marrow from which overall marrow architecture, cellularity and presence of abnormal infiltrates can be reliably determined.

QUANTITATIVE ASPECTS OF ERYTHROPOIESIS

Erythropoiesis is not entirely efficient since about 10–15% of erythropoiesis in a normal bone marrow is ineffective, i.e. the developing erythroblasts die within the marrow and, together with their haemoglobin, they are ingested by marrow macrophages. This ineffective erythropoiesis or 'intramedullary haemolysis' is substantially increased in a number of chronic anaemias — megaloblastic anaemia, myelosclerosis and thalassaemia major being the best examples. Studies with radioactive iron (^{59}Fe) can be used in conjunction with the reticulocyte count and bone marrow appearance to measure the degree of effective and ineffective erythropoiesis. The serum unconjugated bilirubin (derived from breaking-down haemoglobin) and lactate dehydrogenase (LDH, derived from breaking-down cells) are usually raised when ineffective erythropoiesis is marked.

A number of tests can be performed to assess total erythropoiesis, the amount of this that is effective in producing circulating red cells and the lifespan of circulating red cells.

TESTS OF TOTAL ERYTHROPOIESIS

1 *Marrow cellularity and the myeloid : erythroid ratio* (i.e. the proportion of granulocyte precursors to red cell precursors in the bone marrow, normally 2.5 : 1–12 : 1). This ratio falls when total erythropoiesis is selectively increased.
2 *Plasma iron turnover.* The extent of erythropoiesis is assessed firstly by measuring the rate of clearance of transferrin bound ^{59}Fe from the plasma (Fig. 1.19a) and secondly by calculating the plasma iron turnover from the clearance measurement and plasma iron content. As most of the iron normally leaving the plasma is taken up by erythroblasts and reticulocytes, the iron turnover is related to total amount of erythropoietic tissue (effective and ineffective). For example, a plasma iron turnover of three times normal suggests a threefold expansion of erythropoiesis. On the other hand reduced figures suggest erythropoietic hypoplasia.
3 *Carbon monoxide excretion* (only performed as a research procedure).

TESTS OF EFFECTIVE ERYTHROPOIESIS

1 *The reticulocyte count.* This is raised in proportion to the degree of anaemia when erythropoiesis is effective, but is low when there is ineffective erythropoiesis or an abnormality preventing normal marrow response (Table 1.5).
2 *^{59}Fe incorporation into circulating red cells.* The iron incorporated into haemoglobin which reappears in the circulation after the first day of the study is an indication of effective erythropoiesis. This iron has entered erythroblasts and been incorporated into their haemoglobin. Normally 70–80% of the injected ^{59}Fe is

utilised in this manner and reappears in the circulation within ten days (Fig. 1.19a). Maximum red cell iron incorporation values of less than 70% indicate diminished or ineffective erythropoiesis.

The sites of erythropoiesis (medullary and extramedullary) are demonstrated by counting the radioactivity over the sacrum, liver, spleen and heart (Fig. 1.19b).

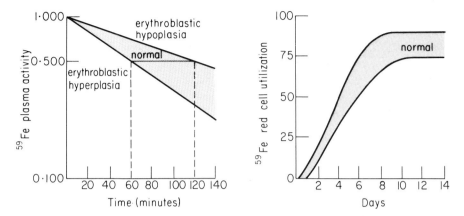

Fig. 1.19a ⁵⁹Fe ferrokinetic study. (*Left*) Initial clearance of ⁵⁹Fe from plasma. This is rapid with a normal half clearance time of 60–140 minutes. Clearance is delayed in erythroblastic hypoplasia and more rapid in erythroblastic hyperplasia. (*Right*) ⁵⁹Fe red cell utilisation or incorporation. In normal subjects this rises steadily from 24 hours to a maximum of 70–80% on the 10–14th day.

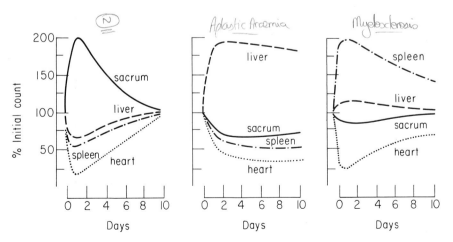

Fig. 1.19b ⁵⁹Fe-ferrokinetic study; surface counting patterns. (*Left*) normal; (*centre*) aplastic anaemia (note lack of accumulation in the bone marrow (sacrum); (*right*) myelosclerosis (pattern of extramedullary erythropoiesis in the liver and spleen).

INEFFECTIVE ERYTHROPOIESIS This implies death of nucleated red cell precursors in the bone marrow. It is particularly marked in megaloblastic anaemia, thalassaemia major and myelosclerosis. It is characterised by excessive bilirubin production, a cellular marrow with a low reticulocyte count, raised serum LDH and hydroxybutyrate dehydrogenase with rapid clearance of injected ^{59}Fe and poor incorporation of this into circulating red cells.

RED CELL LIFESPAN

This is measured by ^{51}Cr-labelled red cell survival. A sample of the subject's blood is incubated with ^{51}Cr which binds firmly to haemoglobin and the labelled cells are re-injected into the circulation. The disappearance of ^{51}Cr from the blood is measured sequentially over the next three weeks. The sites of red cell de-

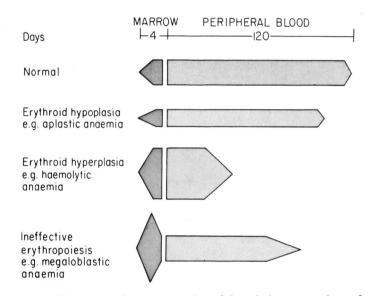

Fig. 1.20 Diagrammatic representation of the relative proportions of marow erythroblastic activity, circulating red cell mass and red cell lifespan in normal subjects and three types of anaemia.

struction are determined by surface counting over the spleen, liver and heart (as an index of blood activity). Typical results in a haemolytic anaemia are shown in Fig. 4.1. Fig. 1.20 shows diagramatically typical changes in marrow erythropoiesis and circulating red cell mass in some of the different types of anaemia.

SELECTED BIBLIOGRAPHY

Brown E.B. (ed.) (1979, 1981, 1983) *Progress in Hematology, XI, XII, XIII*. Grune and Stratton, New York.

Clinics in Haematology (1981) vol. 10.3, *Haematology in Tropical Areas*. Ed. L. Luzzatto. W.B. Saunders, Philadelphia.

Dacie J.V. & Lewis S.M. (1984) *Practical Haematology*, 6th edition. Churchill Livingstone, Edinburgh.

Fairbanks V.F. (ed.) (1983) *Current Hematology*, vol. 2. Wiley Medical, New York.

Hann I.M., Rankin A., Lake B.D. & Pritchard J. (1983) *Colour Atlas of Paediatric Haematology and Oncology*. Oxford Medical Publications, Oxford.

Hardisty R.M. & Weatherall D.J. (eds.) (1982) *Blood and Its Disorders*, 2nd edition. Blackwell Scientific Publications, Oxford.

Harris J.W. & Kellermeyer R.W. (1970) *The Red Cell*. Harvard University Press, Cambridge, Mass.

Hayhoe F.G.T. & Flemans R.J. (1982) *Haematological Cytology*, 2nd edition. Wolfe Medical, London.

Hoffbrand A.V. (ed.) (1981) *Recent Advances in Haematology 3*. Churchill Livingstone, Edinburgh.

Hoffbrand A.V. & Lewis S.M. (eds.) (1981) *Postgraduate Haematology*. Heinemann Medical, London.

MacDonald G.A., Dodds T.C. & Cruickshank B. (1978) *Atlas of Haematology*. Churchill Livingstone, Edinburgh.

Miller *et al* (eds.) (1979) *Smith's Blood Diseases of Infancy and Childhood*, 4th edition. C.V. Mosby, St Louis.

Nathan D.G. & Oski F. (1981) *Hematology of Infancy and Childhood*, 2nd edition. W.B. Saunders, Philadelphia.

Oski F. & Naiman J. L. (1979) *Hematological Problems in the Newborn*, 2nd edition. W.B. Saunders, Philadelphia.

Penington D. *et al* (1978) *de Gruchy's Clinical Haematology in Medical Practice*, 4th edition. Blackwell Scientific Publications, Oxford.

Wickramasinghe S.N. (1975) *Human Bone Marrow*. Blackwell Scientific Publictions, Oxford.

Williams W.J. *et al* (eds.) (1983) *Hematology*, 3rd edition. McGraw-Hill, New York.

Willoughby M.L.N. (1977) *Paediatric Haematology*. Churchill Livingstone, Edinburgh.

Wintrobe M.M. (ed.) (1980) *Blood Pure and Eloquent*. McGraw-Hill, New York.

Wintrobe M.M. *et al* (eds.) (1981) *Clinical Hematology*, 8th edition. Lea & Febiger, Philadelphia.

Zucker Franklyn D. *et al* (1981) *Atlas of Blood Cells*. Lea & Febiger, Philadelphia.

Chapter 2
Iron deficiency and other hypochromic anaemias

Iron deficiency is the commonest cause of anaemia in every country of the world. It is the most important, but not sole, cause of a microcytic, hypochromic anaemia, in which all three red cell indices (the MCV, MCH and MCHC) are reduced and the blood film shows microcytic, hypochromic red cells. This appearance is due to a defect in haemoglobin synthesis (Fig. 2.1). The thalassaemias, in which globin synthesis is reduced, are considered in Chapter 4. Iron deficiency and the hypochromic anaemias other than thalassaemia, and the approach to the diagnosis of a patient found to have a hypochromic anaemia, are discussed in this chapter.

IRON

Nutritional and metabolic aspects

Iron is one of the commonest elements in the earth's crust, yet iron deficiency is the commonest cause of anaemia. This is because the body has limited ability to absorb iron but excess loss of iron due to haemorrhage is frequent.

BODY IRON DISTRIBUTION

Haemoglobin contains about two-thirds of body iron (Table 2.1). It is incorporated from plasma transferrin into developing erythroblasts in the bone marrow and into reticulocytes (Fig. 2.2). Transferrin obtains iron mainly from reticulo-endothelial cells (macrophages). Only a small proportion of plasma iron comes from dietary iron absorbed through the duodenum and jejunum. At the end of their life, red cells are broken down in the macrophages of the RE system and their iron is subsequently released into plasma. Some of the iron is also stored in the RE cells as haemosiderin and ferritin, the amount varying widely according to overall body iron status. *Ferritin* is a water soluble protein-iron complex of mol. wt. 465 000; it is made up of an outer protein

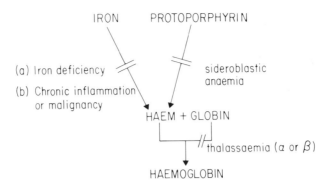

Fig. 2.1 The causes of a hypochromic microcytic anaemia. These include lack of iron (iron deficiency) or of iron release from macrophages to serum (anaemia of chronic inflammation or malignancy), failure of protoporphyrin synthesis (sideroblastic anaemia) or of globin synthesis (α or β-thalassaemia). Lead also inhibits haem and globin synthesis.

shell, apoferritin, consisting of 22 subunits and an iron–phosphate–hydroxide core. It contains up to 20% of its weight as iron and is not visible by light-microscopy. Each molecule of apoferritin may bind up to 4000–5000 atoms of iron and its synthesis is stimulated by iron. *Haemosiderin* is an insoluble protein–iron complex of varying composition containing about 37% of iron by weight. It is probably derived from partial lysosomal digestion of aggregates of ferritin molecules and is visible by light-microscopy after staining by Perls' (Prussian blue) reaction. Iron in ferritin is in the ferric form. It is mobilised after reduction to the ferrous form, vitamin C being involved. A copper-containing enzyme, caeruloplasmin, catalyses oxidation of the iron to the ferric form for binding to plasma transferrin.

Iron is also present in muscle as myoglobin and in most cells of the body in iron-containing enzymes, e.g. cytochromes, succinic dehydrogenase, catalase, etc. (Table 2.1). This tissue iron is less

Table 2.1 The distribution of body iron.

	Amount of iron in average adult		
	Male (g)	Female (g)	% of total
Haemoglobin	2.4	1.7	65
Ferritin and haemosiderin	1.0 (0.3–1.5)	0.3 (0–1.0)	30
Myoglobin	0.15	0.12	3.5
Haem enzymes (e.g. cytochromes, catalase, peroxidases, flavoproteins)	0.02	0.015	0.5
Transferrin-bound iron	0.004	0.003	0.1

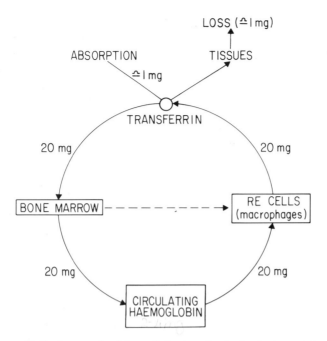

Fig. 2.2 Daily iron cycle. Most of the iron in the body is contained in circulating haemoglobin and is re-utilised for haemoglobin synthesis after the red cells die. Iron is transferred from macrophages to plasma transferrin and so to bone marrow erythroblasts. Iron absorption is normally just sufficient to make up iron loss. Dashed line = ineffective erythropoiesis.

likely to become depleted than haemosiderin, ferritin and haemo-globin in states of iron deficiency, but some reduction of haem-containing enzymes may occur in severe, chronic iron deficiency.

DIETARY IRON

Iron is present in food as ferric hydroxides, ferric–protein complexes and haem–protein complexes. Both the iron content and

Table 2.2 Iron absorption.

Factors favouring	Factors reducing
1 Ferrous form	1 Ferric form
2 Inorganic iron	2 Organic iron
3 Acids — HCl, vitamin C	3 Alkalis — antacids, pancreatic secretions
4 Solubilising agents — e.g. sugars, amino acids	4 Precipitating agents — phytates, phosphates
5 Iron deficiency	5 Iron excess
6 Increased erythropoiesis	6 Decreased erythropoiesis
7 Pregnancy	7 Infection
8 Primary haemachromatosis	8 Tea
	9 Desferrioxamine

proportion of iron absorbed differs from food to food; in general, meat and, in particular, liver is a better source than vegetables, eggs or dairy foods. The average Western diet contains 10–15 mg of iron from which only 5–10% is normally absorbed. The proportion can be increased to 20–30% in iron deficiency or pregnancy (Table 2.2) but, even in these situations, most dietary iron remains unabsorbed.

IRON ABSORPTION

This occurs through the duodenum and less through the jejunum; it is favoured by factors such as acid and reducing agents keeping the iron soluble particularly maintaining it in the Fe^{II} rather than Fe^{III} state (Table 2.2). Organic iron is partly broken down to inorganic iron, but some intact haem iron may also enter the mucosal cell to be split within it. The control of the amount of iron entering portal blood lies partly at the brush borders which influence the amount entering the cell but also within the cell, excess iron being combined with apoferritin to form ferritin which is shed into the gut lumen when the mucosal cell reaches the tip of the intestinal villous. In iron deficiency, more iron enters the cell and a greater proportion of this intramucosal iron is transported into portal blood; in iron overload, less iron enters the cell and a greater proportion of this is shed back into the gut lumen. Iron enters plasma in the Fe^{III} form but, except in rare cases of iron overload, free iron is not present in plasma, since it binds to transferrin in portal blood.

IRON TRANSPORT

Most internal iron exchange is concerned with providing iron to the marrow for erythropoiesis (Fig. 2.2). Iron is transported in plasma bound to a β-globulin, transferrin (siderophyllin), of mol. wt. 80 000. This protein is synthesised in the liver, has a half-life of 8–10 days, and is capable of binding two atoms of iron per molecule. It is re-utilised after it has given up its iron. Normally it is one-third saturated but there is a diurnal variation in serum iron, highest values occurring in the morning and lowest in the evening. Transferrin gains iron mainly from the macrophages of the RE system and it is the diurnal variation in their release of iron which explains the diurnal variation in serum iron concentration. The erythroblasts and reticulocytes (and placenta) obtain iron from transferrin because they have specific receptors for the protein (see Fig. 1.7). Each day, 6 g of haemoglobin are synthesised which requires approximately 20 mg of iron (Fig. 2.2) There is also a minor flow of iron from plasma into non-erythroid cells and it has been estimated that the total plasma iron of only 4 mg turns over seven times each day.

When plasma iron is raised and transferrin is saturated, iron is transferred to parenchymal cells, e.g. those of the liver, endocrine organs, and pancreas, as well as to erythropoietic tissue.

IRON REQUIREMENTS

The amount of iron required each day to compensate for losses from the body and growth varies with age and sex; it is highest in pregnancy and in adolescent and menstruating females (Table 2.3). These groups, therefore, are particularly likely to develop iron deficiency if there is additional iron loss or prolonged reduced intake.

Table 2.3 Estimated daily iron requirements. Units are mg/day.

	Urine, sweat, faeces	Menses	Pregnancy	Growth	Total
Adult male Post-menopausal female	0.5–1				0.5–1
Menstruating female*	0.5–1	0.5–1			1–2
Pregnant female*	0.5–1		1–2		1.5–3.0
Children (average)	0.5			0.6	1
Female (age 12–15)*	0.5–1	0.5–1		0.6	1–2.5

* These groups more likely to develop iron deficiency.

IRON DEFICIENCY

Clinical features

When iron deficiency is developing, the RE stores (haemosiderin and ferritin) become completely depleted before anaemia occurs (Fig. 2.3). At an early stage, there are usually no clinical abnor-

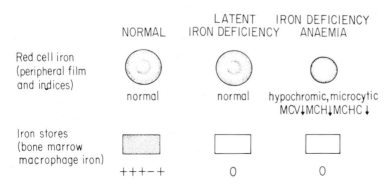

Fig. 2.3 The development of iron deficiency anaemia. Reticuloendothelial (macrophage) stores are lost completely before anaemia develops.

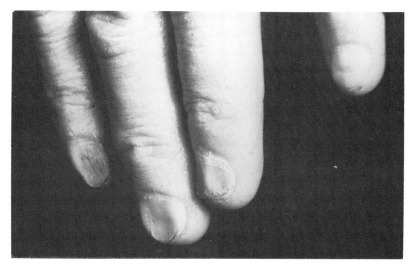

Fig. 2.4 Koilonychia; the typical spoon nails seen in some cases of chronic iron deficiency.

malities the patient may develop the general symptoms and signs of anaemia and also show a painless glossitis, angular stomatitis, brittle, ridged or spoon-nails (koilonychia) (Fig. 2.4), dysphagia due to pharyngeal webs (Paterson–Kelly or Plummer–Vinson syndrome) and unusual dietary cravings (pica). Atrophic gastritis and reduced gastric secretion, usually reversible with iron therapy, occurs in a proportion of patients. The cause of the epithelial cell changes is not clear but may be related to reduction of iron in iron-containing enzymes.

Causes

Chronic blood loss, especially uterine or from the gastrointestinal tract is the dominant cause (Table 2.4). 500 ml of whole blood contains approximately 250 mg of iron and, despite the increased absorption of food iron at an early stage of iron deficiency, negative iron balance is usual in chronic blood loss. Increased demands during infancy, adolescence, pregnancy, lactation and in menstruating women account for the prevalence of latent iron deficiency (absent iron stores without anaemia) and consequent high risk of anaemia in these particular clinical groups. Newborn infants have a store of iron derived from breakdown of excess red cells. From 3 to 6 months, there is a tendency for negative iron balance to occur due to growth. Mixed feeding, particularly with iron-fortified foods, prevents iron deficiency.

In pregnancy, increased iron is needed for an increased maternal red cell mass of about 35%, transfer of 300 mg of iron to the foetus, and because of blood loss at delivery. Although iron absorption is

Table 2.4 Causes of iron deficiency.

---

1 BLOOD LOSS
  Uterine.
  Gastrointestinal. e.g. oesophageal varices, hiatus hernia, peptic ulcer, aspirin ingestion, partial gastrectomy, carcinoma of stomach or caecum, colon or rectum, hookworm, angiodysplasia, colitis, piles, diverticulosis, etc.
  Rarely haematuria, haemoglobinuria, pulmonary haemosiderosis, self-inflicted blood loss.

2 INCREASED DEMANDS (see also Table 2.3)
  Prematurity.
  Growth. ♀, Pregnant ♀ , ♀ (12-15 yrs)
  Child-bearing.

3 MALABSORPTION
  e.g. gastrectomy, coeliac disease.

4 POOR DIET
  A contributory factor in many countries but rarely the sole cause.

---

also increased, prophylactic iron therapy is now given routinely.

Menorrhagia (a loss of 80 ml or more of blood at each cycle) is difficult to assess clinically, although the loss of clots, the use of large numbers of pads or tampons, or prolonged periods all suggest excessive loss.

It has been estimated to take eight years for a normal adult male to develop iron deficiency anaemia solely due to a poor diet or malabsorption causing no iron intake at all and, in clinical practice, inadequate intake or malabsorption are only rarely the sole cause of iron deficiency anaemia. Coeliac disease, partial or total gastrectomy and atrophic gastritis may, however, predispose to iron deficiency. There is also evidence that iron deficiency may cause or contribute to atrophic gastritis. The poor quality, largely vegetable diet taken in many underdeveloped countries may also produce a background of latent iron deficiency on which hookworm, repeated pregnancy and prolonged lactation may place additional stress.

Laboratory findings

These are summarised and contrasted with those in other hypochromic anaemias in Table 2.10.

RED CELL INDICES AND BLOOD FILM. Even before anaemia occurs, the red cell indices fall and they fall progressively as the anaemia becomes more severe. The blood film shows hypochromic, microcytic cells with occasional target cells and pencil-shaped poikilocytes (Fig. 2.5). The reticulocyte count is low in relation to the degree of anaemia. When iron deficiency is associated with severe folate or vitamin B_{12} deficiency a 'dimorphic' film occurs with a dual population of red cells of which one is macrocytic and the other microcytic and hypochromic; the indices may

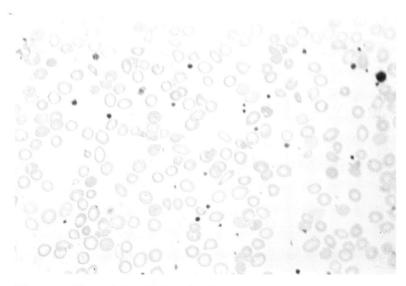

Fig. 2.5 The peripheral blood film in severe iron deficiency anaemia. The cells are microcytic and hypochromic with occasional target cells.

be normal. The platelet count is often moderately raised in iron deficiency, particularly when haemorrhage is continuing.

SERUM IRON AND TOTAL IRON BINDING CAPACITY. The serum iron falls and total iron binding capacity (TIBC) rises to give less than 10% saturation (Fig. 2.6). This contrasts both with the anaemia of chronic disorders (see below) when both the serum iron and the TIBC are reduced and with other hypochromic anaemias where the serum iron is normal or even raised.

BONE MARROW IRON. Bone marrow examination is not essential to assess iron stores except in complicated cases, but iron staining is carried out routinely on all bone marrow aspirations that are performed for any reason. In iron deficiency anaemia there is complete absence of iron from stores (macrophages) and absence of siderotic iron granules from developing erythroblasts. The erythroblasts are small and have a ragged cytoplasm.

SERUM FERRITIN. A small fraction of body ferritin circulates in the serum, the concentration being related to tissue, particularly RE, iron stores. The normal range in men is higher than in women (Table 2.5). In iron deficiency anaemia, the serum ferritin is very low while a raised serum ferritin indicates iron overload or excess release of ferritin from damaged tissues, e.g. acute hepatitis. The serum ferritin is normal or raised in the anaemia of chronic disorders.

Iron deficiency and other hypochromic anaemias   35

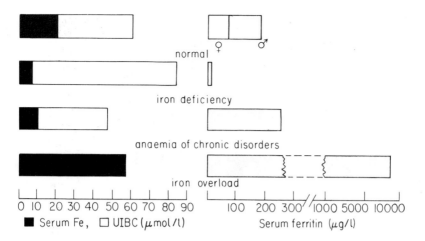

Fig. 2.6 The serum iron, unsaturated serum iron binding capacity (UIBC) and serum ferritin in normal subjects, and in those with iron deficiency, anaemia of chronic disorders and iron overload. The total iron binding capacity (TIBC) is made up by the serum iron and the UIBC. In some laboratories, the transferrin content of serum is measured directly by immunodiffusion, rather than by its ability to bind iron, and is expressed as g/l. Normal serum contains 2–4 g/l of transferrin. (I g/l transferrin≃20 μmol/l binding capacity.)

Table 2.5 Serum ferritin. Units μg/l.

Normal range	
Male	40–340
Female	14–150
Children	7–140
Iron deficiency	0–12
Iron overload	340– > 20 000

FREE ERYTHROCYTE PROTOPORPHYRIN (FEP). This increases early in iron deficiency before anaemia develops. Raised FEP is also found, however, in lead poisoning, some cases of sideroblastic anaemia and in erythropoietic porphyria.

Investigation of the cause of iron deficiency (see also Table 2.4)

In men and post-menopausal women, gastrointestinal blood loss is sought from the clinical history, physical and rectal examination, by occult blood tests, endoscopy and X-rays of the oesophagus,

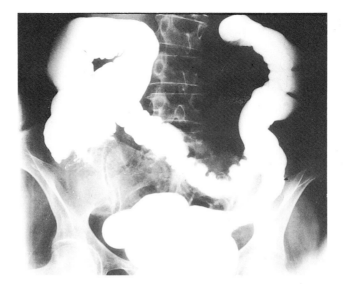

Fig. 2.7 Barium enema of a male patient aged 63 who presented with iron deficiency anaemia. There is a filling defect of the caecum and barium does not enter the terminal ileum. Carcinoma of the caecum was found at laparotomy.

stomach, small and large intestines (Fig. 2.7). Hookworm ova are sought in stools of subjects from areas where this infestation occurs.

NB

Occult blood tests depend on chemical detection of the intact haem ring with guaiac reagents or by the pseudo-peroxidase test. Kits are of varying sensitivity, the more sensitive (e.g. to 2–3 ml daily blood loss) require dietary control of animal haemoproteins to avoid false-positive results while the less sensitive (e.g. to 10–12 ml daily blood loss) may give false-negative results. ^{51}Cr-labelling of red cells with a five day collection of stools is a more accurate method of assessing faecal blood loss.

If these tests are negative and intermittent gastrointestinal blood loss is excluded, loss of iron in the urine as haematuria or haemosiderinuria is considered. A normal chest X-ray excludes the rare condition of pulmonary haemosiderosis. Self-induced haemorrhage is more common in nurses and other medically associated but psychiatrically disturbed individuals. A whole-body counter is useful for demonstrating loss of ^{51}Cr-labelled red cells from the body, without loss in urine or stools. A long-continued poor diet or malabsorption are considered, but are rarely the sole cause of deficiency.

Treatment

The underlying cause is treated as far as possible. In addition, iron is given to correct the anaemia and replenish iron stores.

CORRECTION OF THE DEFICIENCY WITH ORAL IRON. The best preparation is ferrous sulphate which is cheap, contains 67 mg in each 200 mg (anhydrous) tablet and is preferably given in doses spaced by at least 6 hours since the duodenum is refractory to iron absorption for a few hours after a single dose. Optimal absorption is obtained by giving iron fasting but, if side-effects occur, e.g. nausea, abdominal pain, constipation or diarrhoea, these can be reduced by giving iron with food or by using a preparation of lower iron content, e.g. ferrous gluconate, which is also cheap but contains less iron (37 mg) per 300 mg tablet. Ferrous succinate, lactate and fumarate are equally good preparations but more expensive. An elixir is available for children. Combinations of iron with vitamins should not be used (except possibly iron–folic acid combinations in pregnancy) as these are more expensive. Slow-release preparations simply release most of their iron in the lower small intestine from where it cannot be absorbed.

Oral iron therapy should be given for long enough both to correct the anaemia and to replenish body iron stores, which usually means for 4–6 months. The haemoglobin should rise at the rate of about 2 g/dl every 3 weeks. There is a reticulocyte response related to the degree of anaemia. Failure of response to oral iron has several possible causes (Table 2.6) which should all be considered before parenteral iron is used.

Table 2.6 Failure of response to oral iron.

1	Continuing haemorrhage
2	Failure to take tablets
3	Wrong diagnosis — especially thalassaemia trait, sideroblastic anaemia
4	Mixed deficiency — associated folate or vitamin B_{12} deficiency
5	Another cause for anaemia — e.g. malignancy, inflammation
6	Malabsorption — this must be extremely severe
7	Use of slow-release preparation

PROPHYLACTIC IRON THERAPY. This is given throughout pregnancy, often as a single daily tablet combined with folic acid. Patients undergoing regular haemodialysis and premature babies also receive iron prophylactically.

PARENTERAL IRON. This may be given as a total dose infusion of iron–dextran, or by repeated injections of iron–sorbitol–citrate (Jectofer). There may be hypersensitivity or anaphylactoid reactions and parenteral iron is therefore only given when it is considered necessary to replenish body iron rapidly, in, for example, late pregnancy or when oral iron is ineffective (e.g. severe malabsorption) or impractical (e.g. severe gastric or intestinal inflammatory disease). The haematological response to parenteral iron is no faster than to adequate doses of oral iron but the stores are replenished much faster.

Iron overload

A detailed discussion of the causes and clinical and laboratory features of iron overload is beyond the scope of this book. Repeated blood transfusion in patients with chronic refractory anaemias is one important cause of body iron overload (transfusional haemosiderosis). This is most commonly seen in children with beta-thalassaemia major but children with other severe congenital refractory anaemias and adults with acquired sideroblastic anaemia, aplastic anaemia and other unusual anaemias requiring regular blood transfusion may also develop iron overload with damage to the liver, endocrine organs and heart. In some refractory anaemias with increased ineffective erythropoiesis, iron loading occurs after many years from excess absorption, even in the absence of blood transfusions, e.g. in some cases of thalassaemia intermedia and sideroblastic anaemia. The methods of assessing iron stores and tissue damage due to excessive iron are summarised in Table 2.7. The management of this life-threatening situation is discussed on p. 78.

Table 2.7 Iron overload.

Methods of assessment of iron stores
Serum ferritin
Serum iron and percentage saturation of transferrin (iron-binding capacity)
Bone marrow biopsy (reticulo-endothelial stores)
Liver biopsy (parenchymal and reticulo-endothelial stores)
Liver CT scan
Desferrioxamine excretion test (chelatable iron)
Repeated phlebotomy until iron deficiency occurs.

Assessment of tissue damage due to iron overload
Cardiac: clinical, chest X-ray, ECG, echocardiography
Liver: liver function tests, liver biopsy
Endocrine: glucose tolerance test, pituitary gonadotrophin release test, etc.

ANAEMIA OF CHRONIC DISORDERS

One of the most common anaemias occurs in patients with a variety of chronic inflammatory and malignant diseases (Table 2.8). The characteristic features are: 1. normochromic, normocytic or mildly hypochromic indices and red cell morphology; 2. mild and non-progressive anaemia (haemoglobin rarely less than 9.0 g/dl)—the severity being related to the severity of the disease; 3. both the serum iron and TIBC are reduced; 4. the serum ferritin is normal or raised, and 5. bone marrow storage (RE) iron is normal but erythroblast iron is reduced (Table 2.10).

Table 2.8 Causes of the anaemia of chronic disorders.

1 *Chronic inflammatory diseases*
   a infections, e.g. pulmonary abscess, tuberculosis, osteomyelitis, pneumonia, bacterial endocarditis
   b non-infectious, e.g. rheumatoid arthritis, SLE and other connective tissue diseases, sarcoid, Crohn's disease
2 *Malignant diseases*
   e.g. carcinoma, lymphoma, sarcoma

The pathogenesis of this anaemia appears to be related to the decreased release of iron from macrophages to plasma, reduced red cell lifespan and an inadequate erythropoietin response to anaemia. The anaemia is only corrected by successful treatment of the underlying disease but does not respond to iron therapy despite the low serum iron. In many conditions this anaemia is complicated by anaemia due to other causes, e.g. iron, vitamin B_{12} or folate deficiency, renal failure, bone marrow failure, hypersplenism, endocrine abnormality, etc. and these are discussed on p. 94.

SIDEROBLASTIC ANAEMIA

This is a refractory anaemia with hypochromic cells in the peripheral blood and increased marrow iron with many pathological ring sideroblasts present (Fig. 2.8). These are abnormal erythroblasts containing numerous iron granules arranged in a ring or collar around the nucleus instead of the few randomly distributed iron granules seen when normal erythroblasts are stained for iron. The anaemia is classified into different types (Table 2.9). There is probably always a defect in haem synthesis. In the hereditary forms, the anaemia is characterised by a markedly hypochromic and microcytic blood picture. This is due to a congenital enzyme defect, e.g. of delta-amino-laevulinic acid synthetase or haem synthetase. The primary acquired form, which occurs in either sex mainly in middle and old age, is due to a somatic mutation of the erythroid progenitor cells causing not only defects in haem synthesis but also defects in DNA synthesis with megaloblastic and other dyserythro-

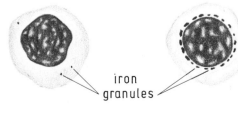

iron
granules

Normal
sideroblast

Ring
sideroblast

Fig. 2.8 A normal erythroblast and a ring sideroblast stained for iron. The normal contains 2 or 3 granules, randomly distributed. In the ring sideroblast there are many granules arranged around the nucleus.

Table 2.9 Classification of sideroblastic anaemia.

[handwritten left margin: Microcytic Hypochromic]

[handwritten: ↑ MCV]

Hereditary	usually occurs in males, transmitted by females; also occurs rarely in females
Acquired	**a** primary *– myelodysplastic Syndromes .*
	b associated with malignant diseases of the bone marrow: e.g. myelodysplastic syndromes, myelosclerosis, myeloid leukaemia, myeloma
	c secondary—drugs—e.g. antituberculous (isoniazid, *∝ B6 antagonist* cycloserine), alcohol, lead

poietic features and frequently a raised MCV. This form sometimes transforms into acute myeloblastic leukaemia after many years of follow-up and has been classified with the myelodysplastic syndromes (p. 150).

In the hereditary and primary acquired diseases, 50% or more of marrow erythroblasts are ring sideroblasts. Ring sideroblasts also occur with lesser frequency in other marrow disorders, especially the myeloproliferative and myelodysplastic syndromes (see p. 150) and myeloma. They may also occur in the bone marrow of patients taking certain drugs, excess alcohol or with lead poisoning (Table 2.9). Vitamin B_6 (pyridoxine) deficiency or vitamin B_6 antagonists (e.g. isoniazid) are rare causes. In some patients, there is a response to pyridoxine therapy. Folate deficiency may occur and folic acid therapy should also be tried. In many severe cases, however, repeated blood transfusions are the only method of maintaining a satisfactory haemoglobin concentration and transfusional iron overload becomes a major problem.

Lead poisoning

Lead inhibits both haem and globin synthesis at a number of points. In addition it interferes with breakdown of RNA by inhibiting the enzyme pyrimidine 5′ nucleotidase, causing accumulation of denatured RNA in red cells, the RNA giving an appearance called punctate basophilia on the ordinary (Romanowsky) stain (Fig. 1.17b). The anaemia may be hypochromic or predominantly haemolytic, and the bone marrow may show ring sideroblasts. Free erythrocyte protoporphyin is raised.

Differential diagnosis of a hypochromic anaemia

Table 2.10 lists the laboratory investigations that may be necessary. The clinical history is particularly important as the source of the haemorrhage leading to iron deficiency or the presence of a chronic disease may be revealed. The country of origin and the family history may suggest a possible diagnosis of thalassaemia or other haemoglobinopathy. Physical examination may also be helpful in determining a site of haemorrhage, features of a chronic inflam-

Table 2.10 Laboratory diagnosis of a hypochromic anaemia.

	Iron deficiency	Chronic inflammation or malignancy	Thalassaemia trait (α or β)	Sideroblastic anaemia
MCV MCH MCHC*	All reduced in relation to severity of anaemia	Low normal or mild reduction	All reduced very low for degree of anaemia	Very low in congenital type but MCV often raised in acquired type
Serum iron	reduced	reduced	normal	raised
TIBC	raised	reduced	normal	normal
Serum ferritin	reduced	normal	normal	raised
Bone marrow iron stores	absent	present	present	present
Erythroblast iron	absent	absent	present	ring forms
Haemoglobin electrophoresis	normal	normal	Hb A$_2$ raised in β form†	normal

* With modern electronic counters, the MCHC is not a reliable index of a hypochromic anaemia.
† Other types including major forms (see Chapter 4).

matory or malignant disease, koilonychia, or, in some haemoglobinopathies, an enlarged spleen or bony deformities.

The red cells tend to be particularly small often with an MCV of 60 fl or less even when anaemia is mild or even absent in thalassaemia trait, the red cell count being over 5.0×10^{12}/l. On the other hand, in iron deficiency anaemia the indices fall progressively with the degree of anaemia, and when anaemia is mild the indices are often only just reduced below normal (e.g. MCV 75–80 fl). In the anaemia of chronic disorders, the indices are also not markedly low, with an MCV in the range 75–82 fl being usual.

It is usual to perform a serum iron and TIBC measurement or alternatively serum ferritin estimation to confirm a diagnosis of iron deficiency. Haemoglobin electrophoresis with estimation of haemoglobins A$_2$ and F is carried out in all patients suspected of thalassaemia or a haemoglobinopathy because of the family history, country of origin and red cell indices and blood film. Obviously iron deficiency or the anaemia of chronic disorders may occur in these subjects. Beta-thalassaemia trait is characterised by a raised haemoglobin A$_2$ percentage above 3.5, but in alpha-thalassaemia trait there is no abnormality on simple haemoglobin studies and the diagnosis is usually made by exclusion of all other causes of hypochromic red cells and by globin chain synthesis studies. In some patients, however, occasional red cells show deposits of HbH (β^4) in reticulocyte preparations. Bone marrow examination is essential if a diagnosis of sideroblastic anaemia is suspected but is not usually needed in diagnosis of the other hypochromic anaemias.

The investigation of a hypochromic anaemia is not complete if a diagnosis of iron deficiency is confirmed. It is then mandatory to determine the cause of the deficiency — in nearly every case chronic haemorrhage. In females of childbearing age, uterine haemorrhage is the frequent cause but in males and post-menopausal females the gastrointestinal tract is the usual source of bleeding and faecal occult blood tests, endoscopy, barium meal, follow-through and enema X-rays, tests for hookworm ova and, in rare cases, coeliac axis angiography may be needed. ^{51}Cr-labelled red cells may be used to quantify stool blood loss.

SELECTED BIBLIOGRAPHY

Beris P., Graf J. & Micscher P.A. (1983) Primary acquired sideroblastic and primary acquired refractory anemia. *Seminars in Hematology,* **20,** 101–13.

Bothwell T.H., Charlton R.W., Cook J.D. & Finch C.A. (1980) *Iron Metabolism in Man.* Blackwell Scientific Publications, Oxford.

Charlton R.W. & Bothwell T.H. (1983) Iron absorption. *Annual Review of Medicine* **34,** 55–68.

Clinics in Haematology (1982) vol 11.2, *Disorders of Iron Metabolism.* Ed A. Jacobs. W.B. Saunders, Philadelphia.

Jacobs A. (1981) Disorders of iron metabolism. In *Recent Advances in Haematology 3*, ed. A.V. Hoffbrand. Churchill Livingstone, Edinburgh.

Jacobs A. & Worwood M. (eds.) (1980) *Iron in Biochemistry and Medicine*, 2nd edition. Academic Press, London.

Lee G.R. (1983) The anemia of chronic disease. *Seminars in Hematology,* **20,** 61–8.

Methods in Haematology (1980) *Iron,* vol. 1, ed. J.D. Cook. Churchill Livingstone, Edinburgh.

Major textbooks of haematology (see Chapter 1).

Chapter 3
Megaloblastic anaemia and other macrocytic anaemias

MEGALOBLASTIC ANAEMIA

This is a group of anaemias in which the erythroblasts in the bone marrow show a characteristic abnormality, maturation of the nucleus being delayed relative to that of the cytoplasm. The nuclear chromatin maintains an open, stippled, lacey appearance despite normal haemoglobin formation in the erythroblasts as they mature. The underlying defect accounting for the asynchronous maturation of the nucleus is defective DNA synthesis and, in clinical practice, this is usually due to deficiency of vitamin B_{12} or folate but, less commonly, abnormalities of metabolism of these

Table 3.1 Causes of megaloblastic anaemia.

1 Vitamin B_{12} deficiency
2 Folate deficiency
3 Abnormalities of vitamin B_{12} or folate metabolism
4 Other defects of DNA synthesis
   a congenital enzyme deficiencies
   b acquired, e.g. therapy with hydroxyurea, cytosine arabinoside

vitamins or other lesions in DNA synthesis may cause an identical haematological appearance (Table 3.1). Before considering the anaemia, dietary and metabolic aspects of the two vitamins are reviewed.

Vitamin B_{12}

This vitamin is synthesised in nature by micro-organisms and animals acquire it by eating other animal foods, by internal production due to intestinal bacteria (not in humans) or by eating bacterially contaminated foods. The vitamin consists of a small group of compounds, the cobalamins, which have the same basic structure with a cobalt atom at the centre of a corrin ring which is attached to a nucleotide portion (Fig. 3.1). Methyl (CH_3) and ado (deoxadenosyl) groups are attached to the cobalt in the two main

44

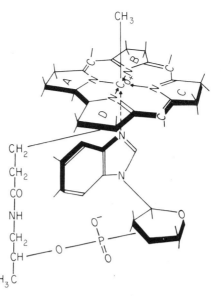

Fig. 3.1   The structure of methylcobalamin (methyl B_{12}), the main form of vitamin B_{12} in human plasma. Other forms include deoxyadenosylcobalamin (ado B_{12}), the main form in human tissues; hydroxocobalamin (hydroxo B_{12}), the main form in treatment; and cyanocobalamin (cyano B_{12}), the form used radioactively labelled ([57]Co or [58]Co) to study vitamin B_{12} absorption or metabolism.

natural forms, while cyano (CN) and hydroxo (OH) groups are present in the two more stable pharmacological forms (Fig. 3.1). The vitamin is found in foods of animal origin such as liver, fish and dairy produce but does not occur in fruit, cereals or vegetables unless these have been contaminated by bacteria.

A normal diet contains a large excess of vitamin B_{12} (B_{12}) compared with daily needs. B_{12} is released from protein complexes in food, combined with the glycoprotein intrinsic factor (IF), synthesised by the gastric parietal cells and the complex is then attached to ileal surface receptors (Fig. 3.2). B_{12} is absorbed into portal blood where it appears attached to a plasma binding protein, transcobalamin II (T C II) which delivers it to bone marrow and other tissues. Intrinsic factor itself is not absorbed. Most B_{12} in plasma, however, is tightly bound to another transport protein, transcobalamin I (T C I), which is thought to be largely synthesised by granulocytes. In myeloproliferative diseases where granulocyte production is greatly increased, the TCI and B_{12} levels in serum may rise considerably. B_{12} bound to TCI does not transfer readily to marrow; it appears to be functionally 'dead'.

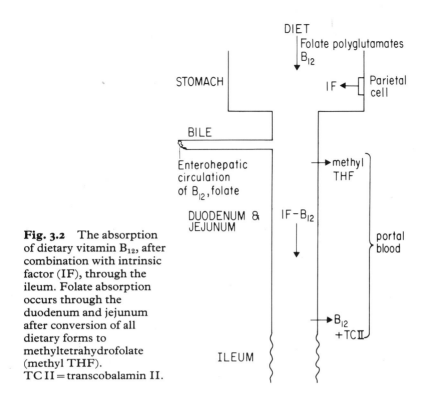

Fig. 3.2 The absorption of dietary vitamin B_{12}, after combination with intrinsic factor (IF), through the ileum. Folate absorption occurs through the duodenum and jejunum after conversion of all dietary forms to methyltetrahydrofolate (methyl THF). TC II = transcobalamin II.

Table 3.2 Vitamin B_{12} and folate: nutritional aspects.

	Vitamin B_{12}	Folate
Normal dietary intake	7–30 μg	600–1000 μg
Main foods	Animal produce only	Most, especially liver, greens and yeast
Cooking	little effect	easily destroyed
Minimal daily requirement	1–2 μg	100–200 μg
Body stores	2–3 mg (3–5mg). (sufficient for 2–4 years)	10–12 mg (sufficient for 4 months)
Absorption—		
site	ileum	duodenum and jejunum
mechanism	intrinsic factor	conversion to methyltetrahydrofolate
limit	2–3 μg daily	50–80% of dietary content
Major intracellular physiological forms	methyl- and adenosyl-cobalamin	reduced polyglutamate derivatives
Usual therapeutic form	hydroxocobalamin	Folic (pteroylglutamic) acid

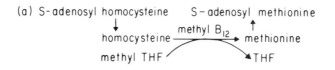

(a) S-adenosyl homocysteine   S-adenosyl methionine

homocysteine $\xrightarrow{\text{methyl } B_{12}}$ methionine

methyl THF   THF

(b) propionyl CoA → methylmalonyl CoA $\xrightarrow{\text{ado } B_{12}}$ succinyl CoA

Fig. 3.3 The biochemical reactions of vitamin B_{12} in humans.

$\times$ B_{12} is coenzyme for two biochemical reactions in the body: firstly as methyl B_{12} in the methylation of homocysteine to methionine by methyl THF (Fig. 3.3a) and secondly as adenosyl B_{12} (ado-B_{12}) in conversion of methylmalonyl CoA to succinyl CoA (Fig. 3.3b).

Folate

Folic (pteroylglutamic) acid is yellow, stable and water soluble. It is the parent compound of a large group of compounds, the folates, which are derived from it by 1. addition of extra glutamic acid residues, so-called pteroyl- or folate-polyglutamates, 2. reduction to di- or the metabolically active tetrahydro-folates, and 3. addition of single carbon units, e.g. methyl (CH_3—), formyl (CHO—) or methylene (=CH_2) (Fig. 3.4). Human beings are unable to synthesise the folate structure and thus require preformed

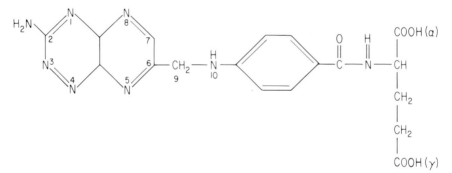

Fig. 3.4 The structure of pteroylglutamic acid (folic acid). Dietary folates may contain: i Additional hydrogen atoms at positions 7 & 8 (dihydrofolate) or 5,6,7, & 8 (tetrahydrofolate); ii a formyl group at N_5 or N_{10} or a methyl group at N_5; iii additional glutamate moieties attached to the gamma carboxyl group of the glutamate moiety.

folate as a vitamin. Bacteria synthesise folate *de novo* from pteridine, para-amino benzoic acid and glutamic acid. Sulphonamides block the incorporation of para-amino benzoic acid and thus inhibit bacterial folate synthesis.

$\times$ Folate polyglutamates are the main intracellular forms but, in body fluids, folate is transported as the mono-glutamate methyl THF—loosely bound to proteins. During absorption through the
Albumin

upper small intestine, all dietary forms are converted to methyl THF (Fig. 3.5). Folates are needed in a variety of biochemical reactions in the body involving single carbon unit transfer. Three of these are in DNA synthesis, two in the synthesis of purines and the third in pyrimidine synthesis in the key reaction—thymidylate synthetase (Fig. 3.5.). The other folate-dependent reactions are largely concerned in amino acid interconversions.

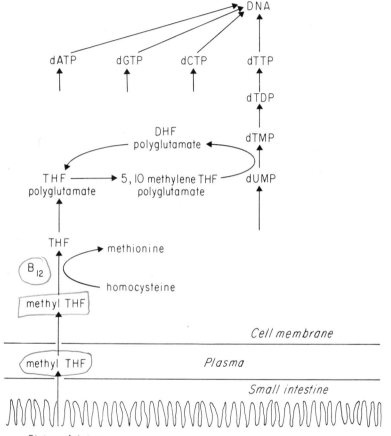

Fig. 3.5 The biochemical basis of megaloblastic anaemia due to vitamin B_{12} or folate deficiency. Folate is required as its coenzyme form 5,10 methylene tetrahydrofolate polyglutamate in the synthesis of thymidine monophosphate from its precursor deoxyuridine monophosphate. Vitamin B_{12} is needed to convert methyl tetrahydrofolate, which enters cells from plasma, to tetrahydrofolate, from which polyglutamate forms of folate are synthesised. Dietary folates are all converted to methyl tetrahydrofolate (a monoglutamate) by the small intestine. THF = tetrahydrofolate, DHF = dihydrofolate, B_{12} = Vitamin B_{12}, d = deoxyribose, U = uracil, T = thymine, C = cytosine, G = guanine, A = adenine, MP = monophosphate, DP = diphosphate, TP = triphosphate.

Biochemical basis for megaloblastic anaemia

Folate deficiency is thought to cause megaloblastic anaemia by inhibiting thymidylate synthesis, a rate-limiting step in DNA synthesis in which one of the two pyrimidine bases, thymine, is synthesised (Fig. 3.5). This reaction needs 5,10 methylene THF polyglutamate as coenzyme. Vitamin B_{12}, by its involvement in homocysteine methylation to methionine, is needed in the conversion of methyl THF to THF which is the likely substrate for folate polyglutamate synthesis. The folate polyglutamates act as intracellular coenzymes including 5,10 methylene THF polyglutamate, the coenzyme form of folate involved in the thymidylate synthetase reaction (Fig. 3.5). Lack of vitamin B_{12}, therefore, 'traps' folate as its transport methyl THF form and deprives cells of the 5,10 methylene THF polyglutamate form needed for DNA synthesis. Other congenital or acquired causes of megaloblastic anaemia (e.g. antimetabolite drugs) inhibit purine or pyrimidine synthesis at one or other step.

During thymidylate synthesis, folate becomes oxidised to functionally dead dihydrofolate (DHF) polyglutamate (Fig. 3.5). Regeneration of active tetrahydrofolate polyglutamate requires the enzyme, dihydrofolate reductase. Inhibitors of this enzyme (e.g. methotrexate) therefore inhibit DNA synthesis and are useful drugs mainly in the treatment of malignant disease. The weaker antagonist, pyrimethamine is used primarily against malaria, and trimethoprim, active against bacterial dihydrofolate reductase, is used in the antibacterial combination with a sulphonamide, as co-trimoxazole. Toxicity due to methotrexate or pyrimethamine is reversed by giving the patient the stable fully reduced folate, folinic acid (5-formyltetrahydrofolate).

Vitamin B_{12} deficiency

In Western countries, the deficiency is usually due to (Addisonian) pernicious anaemia (Table 3.3). Much less commonly veganism in which the diet lacks B_{12} (usually in Hindu Indians), gastrectomy or small intestinal lesions may cause the deficiency. There is no syndrome of B_{12} deficiency due to increased utilisation or loss of the vitamin so the deficiency inevitably takes at least 2 years to develop, i.e. the time needed for body stores to deplete at the rate of 1–2 μg each day when there is no new B_{12} entering the body from the diet. Nitrous oxide, however, may rapidly inactivate body B_{12} (p. 58).

PERNICIOUS ANAEMIA (PA)

The common adult form consists of atrophy of the stomach, probably auto-immune in origin. The wall of the stomach is thin, with a plasma cell and lymphoid infiltrate of the lamina propria. There

Table 3.3 Causes of vitamin B_{12} deficiency.

1 VEGANISM
2 MALABSORPTION
    gastric causes
    Adult (Addisonian) pernicious anaemia
    Congenital lack of IF
    Total or partial gastrectomy
    intestinal causes
    Intestinal stagnant loop syndrome — jejunal diverticulosis, blind-loop, stricture, etc.
    Chronic tropical sprue
    Ileal resection and Crohn's disease
    Congenital selective malabsorption with proteinuria

Note Other causes of malabsorption of B_{12} (e.g. fish tapeworm, severe pancreatitis, coeliac disease, therapy with metformin, phenformin) do not usually lead to clinically important B_{12} deficiency.

is achlorhydria and secretion of IF is absent or almost absent. Corticosteroid therapy can improve the gastric lesion with a return of acid secretion but, because of the side-effects, PA is not treated in this way.

More females than males are affected (1.6:1) with a peak age occurrence of 60, and there may be associated auto-immune disease, e.g. myxoedema, thyroiditis, adrenal atrophy, vitiligo, hypoparathyroidism, diabetes and hypogammaglobulinaemia. The disease (most common in northern Europeans but found in all races) tends to occur in families and there is an association with blood group A, blue eyes and early greying, and there is an increased incidence of carcinoma of the stomach (about 2–3% of all cases of PA). There is no overall association with any HLA antigens. Ninety per cent of patients show parietal cell antibody in the serum, and 50% an antibody to IF (Type I or blocking) which inhibits IF binding to B_{12}. Thirty-five per cent show a second (Type II or precipitating) antibody to IF which inhibits its ileal binding site. IF antibodies are virtually specific for PA but occur in the serum of only half the patients whereas the more common parietal cell antibody is less specific and occurs quite commonly in older subjects (e.g. 16% of normal women over 60). Both types of antibody may also occur in gastric juice. If present, IF antibody inhibits the function of small amounts of remaining IF in gastric juice and this may contribute to the malabsorption of vitamin B_{12}.

Childhood PA consists either of congenital lack or abnormality of IF (with an otherwise normal stomach and normal acid secretion) or an early onset of the adult, auto-immune form. Congenital lack of IF usually presents at about 2 years of age when stores of B_{12} which were derived from the mother *in utero* have been used up.

Folate deficiency

This is most often due to a poor dietary intake of folate alone or in combination with a condition of increased folate utilisation or malabsorption (Table 3.4). Excess cell turnover of any sort, including pregnancy, is the main cause of increased need for folate. The mechanism by which anticonvulsants and barbiturates cause the deficiency is still controversial.

Table 3.4   Causes of folate deficiency.

1	NUTRITIONAL—especially old age, poverty, scurvy, partial gastrectomy, goat's milk anaemia, etc.
2	MALABSORPTION—tropical sprue, coeliac disease (adult or child). Possible contributory factor to folate deficiency in some patients with: partial gastrectomy, extensive jejunal resection, Crohn's disease
3	EXCESS UTILISATION
	a *Physiological:* pregnancy and lactation, prematurity
	b *Pathological:* haematological diseases—haemolytic anaemias, myelosclerosis; malignant disease—carcinoma, lymphoma, myeloma; inflammatory diseases—Crohn's disease, tuberculosis, rheumatoid arthritis, psoriasis, exfoliative dermatitis
4	EXCESS URINARY FOLATE LOSS—active liver disease, congestive heart failure
5	ANTICONVULSANT DRUG THERAPY
6	MIXED—liver disease, alcoholism, intensive care

Clinical features of megaloblastic anaemia

The onset is usually insidious with gradually progressive symptoms and signs of anaemia (Chapter 2). Sometimes an intermittent infection causes the patient to seek medical help. The patient may be mildly jaundiced (lemon yellow tint) from the excess breakdown of haemoglobin mainly due to increased ineffective erythropoiesis but also to shortened red cell survival. Glossitis (a beefy red, sore tongue, Fig. 3.6), angular stomatitis and mild symptoms of malabsorption with loss of weight may be present due to the epithelial abnormality. Purpura due to thrombocytopenia and widespread melanin pigmentation are less frequent presenting features. Many symptomless patients are diagnosed when a blood count that has been performed for another reason reveals macrocytosis.

VITAMIN B_{12} NEUROPATHY (SUBACUTE COMBINED DEGENERATION OF THE CORD)

Severe B_{12} deficiency may cause a progressive neuropathy affecting the peripheral sensory nerves, and posterior and lateral columns (Fig. 3.7). The neuropathy is symmetrical and affects

Table 3.5 Definite effects of vitamin B_{12} or folate deficiency.

1 Megaloblastic anaemia
2 Macrocytosis of epithelial cell surfaces
3 Neuropathy (for vitamin B_{12} only)
4 Sterility
5 Rarely, reversible melanin skin pigmentation

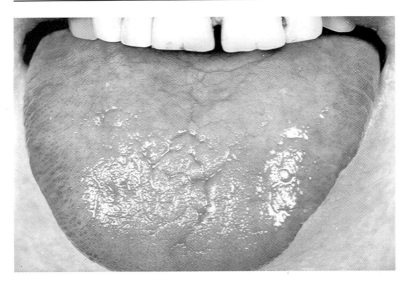

Fig. 3.6 The tongue in a patient with megaloblastic anaemia. Note the beefy appearance.

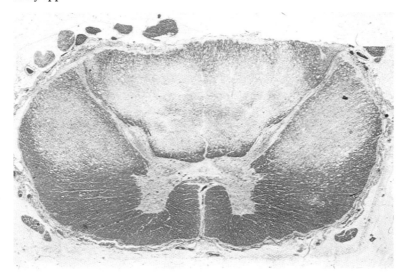

Fig. 3.7 A cross-section of the spinal cord in a patient who died with subacute combined degeneration of the cord (Weigert-Pal stain). There is demyelination of dorsal and dorso-lateral columns.

the lower limbs more than upper. The patient, more often male, notices tingling in the feet, difficulty in walking and may fall over in the dark. Rarely, optic atrophy or severe psychiatric symptoms are present. Anaemia may be severe, mild or even absent, but the blood film and bone marrow appearances are always abnormal. Recent work suggests the neuropathy may be due to lack of s-adenosyl methionine synthesis (see Fig. 3.3) with a defect in methylation reactions needed for myelin formation.

Laboratory findings in megaloblastic anaemia

The anaemia is macrocytic (MCV > 95 fl and often as high as 120–140 fl in severe cases) and the macrocytes are typically oval in shape (Fig. 3.8). The reticulocyte count is low in relation to the degree of anaemia and the total white cell and platelet counts may be moderately reduced, especially in severely anaemic patients. A proportion of the neutrophils show hypersegmented nuclei (nuclei with 6 or more lobes). The bone marrow is usually hypercellular

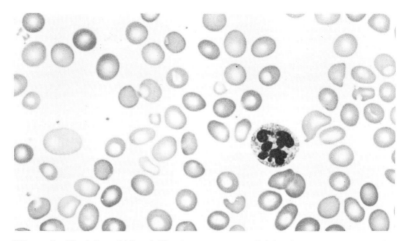

Fig. 3.8 Peripheral blood film in severe megaloblastic anaemia. Note the oval macrocytes and hypersegmented neutrophil.

and the erythroblasts are large and show failure of nuclear maturation maintaining an open, fine, primitive chromatin pattern but normal haemoglobinisation (Fig. 3.9). Many dying erythroblasts may be seen. Giant and abnormally shaped metamyelocytes are present. The changes correlate with the severity of anaemia so that, in mildly anaemic patients, the abnormalities may be quite difficult to recognise.

The serum unconjugated bilirubin, hydroxybutyrate and LDH are all raised (due to marrow cell breakdown — ineffective erythropoesis and leucopoiesis). The serum iron and ferritin may be normal or raised.

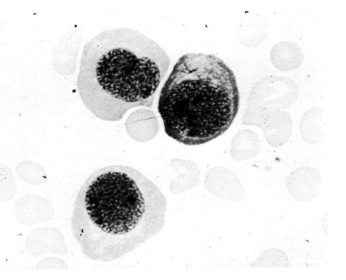

Fig. 3.9 Megaloblasts in the bone marrow in a patient with severe megaloblastic anaemia. Note the fine, open, stippled (primitive) appearance of the nuclear chromatin even in late cells (pale cytoplasm and some haemoglobin formation).

DIAGNOSIS OF VITAMIN B_{12} OR FOLATE DEFICIENCY

It is usual to assay serum B_{12}, serum and red cell folate (Table 3.6). Either microbiological or radioisotope dilution assays are used. The serum B_{12} is usually very low in megaloblastic anaemia or neuropathy due to B_{12} deficiency. The serum and red cell folate are both low in megaloblastic anaemia due to folate deficiency; in B_{12} deficiency the serum folate tends to rise but the red cell folate falls due to failure of folate polyglutamate synthesis. In the absence of B_{12} deficiency, however, the red cell folate is a more accurate guide than the serum folate of tissue folate status. Combined deficiencies may be difficult to sort out. The haematological response of the patient to specific therapy is particularly helpful in these cases with low serum levels of both vitamins providing that daily physiological doses (1 μg B_{12} or 100 μg folic acid) are used since a response will

Table 3.6 Laboratory tests for vitamin B_{12} and folate deficiency.

Test	Normal value	Result in	
		Vitamin B_{12} deficiency	Folate deficiency
Serum B_{12}	160–925 ng/l	Low	Normal or borderline
Serum folate	3.0–15.0 μg/l	Normal or raised	Low
Red cell folate	160–640 μg/l	Normal or low	Low

only occur if there is deficiency of the appropriate vitamin. Large doses of folic acid (e.g. 5 mg daily) cause a haematological response (but may aggravate the neuropathy) in B_{12} deficiency and thus should not be given alone unless B_{12} deficiency has been excluded, e.g. by showing a normal serum B_{12} level.

Excretion of methylmalonic acid has been used as a test for B_{12} deficiency, and excretion of forminoglutamic acid (Figlu) as a test for folate deficiency but neither is now used in routine practice.

The deoxyuridine suppression test is, however, used in certain specialised laboratories. It measures the degree to which unlabelled deoxyuridine suppresses uptake of radioactive thymidine into DNA of bone marrow cells *in vitro*, and is an indirect measure of thymidylate synthesis. The test is abnormal (less suppression) in megaloblastic anaemia due to B_{12} or folate deficiency, and it can be corrected *in vitro* with addition of the appropriate vitamin.

TESTS FOR CAUSES OF DEFICIENCIES (Table 3.7)

For B_{12} deficiency, absorption tests using an oral dose of radioactive cobalt (^{58}Co or ^{57}Co)-labelled cyanocobalamin are valuable in distinguishing malabsorption from an inadequate diet and, when the test is repeated with an active IF preparation, in distinguishing a gastric lesion such as pernicious anaemia, when IF corrects labelled B_{12} absorption, from an intestinal lesion, when additional IF does not correct the test (Table 3.8). Absorption is most frequently measured indirectly by the urinary excretion (Schilling) technique in which absorbed labelled B_{12} is 'flushed' into a 24 hour urine sample by a large (1000 μg) dose of non-radioactive B_{12} given simultaneously with the labelled oral dose. Whole body counting, faecal excretion, plasma counting and hepatic counting techniques are also used in some centres.

Other useful tests are listed in Table 3.7. These are mainly concerned with assessing gastric function and testing for antibodies to gastric antigens. In all cases of pernicious anaemia, X-ray or endoscopy studies should be performed to confirm the presence of gastric atrophy and exclude carcinoma of the stomach.

For folate deficiency, the diet history is most important,

Table 3.7 Tests for cause of vitamin B_{12} or folate deficiency.

Vitamin B_{12}	*Folate*
1 Diet history	1 Diet history
2 B_{12} absorption ± IF	2 Tests for intestinal
3 IF, parietal cell antibodies	malabsorption
4 Endoscopy or barium meal	3 Jejunal biopsy
and follow-through	4 Underlying disease
5 Gastric function — acid, IF	

Table 3.8 Results of absorption tests of radioactive B_{12}.

	Dose of labelled B_{12} given alone	Dose of labelled B_{12} given with I F
Vegan	normal	normal
Pernicious anaemia or gastrectomy	low	normal
Ileal lesion	low	low
Intestinal blind-loop syndrome	low*	low*

* Corrected by antibiotic therapy.

although it is difficult to estimate folate intake accurately. Unsuspected coeliac disease or other underlying conditions (see Table 3.4) should also be considered.

Treatment

Most cases only need therapy with the appropriate vitamin (Table 3.9). In severely anaemic patients in whom there is no clear indication which deficiency is present but who need treatment urgently, it may be safer to initiate treatment with both vitamins. In the elderly, the presence of heart failure should be corrected with diuretics and oral potassium supplements given for 10 days (since hypokalaemia has been found to occur during the response in some cases). Infection should be sought and treated. Blood transfusion should be avoided since it may cause circulatory overload. If it is essential (because of anoxia) 1–2 units of packed cells should be given slowly, possibly with removal of blood from the other arm.

Table 3.9 Treatment of megaloblastic anaemia.

	Vitamin B_{12} deficiency	Folate deficiency
Compound	*Hydroxocobalamin*	*Folic acid*
Route	Intramuscular	Oral
Dose	1000 μg	5 mg
Initial	6 × 1000 μg over 2–3 weeks	Daily for 4 months
Maintenance	1000 μg every 3 months	Depends on underlying disease. Life-long therapy may be needed in chronic inherited haemolytic anaemias, myelosclerosis, renal dialysis.
Prophylactic	Total gastrectomy Ileal resection	Pregnancy, severe haemolytic anaemias, dialysis, prematurity

RESPONSE TO THERAPY. The patient feels better after 24–48 hours of correct vitamin therapy with increased appetite and well being. A reticulocyte response begins on the 2nd or 3rd day with a peak at 6–7 days — its height is inversely proportional to the initial red cell count (Fig. 3.10). The haemoglobin should rise by 2–3 g/dl each fortnight. The white cell and platelet counts become normal in 7–10 days and the marrow is normoblastic in about 48 hours, although giant metamyelocytes persist for up to 12 days. The serum iron falls over the first day and the LDH and ferritin more slowly.

The peripheral neuropathy may partly improve but spinal cord damage is irreversible.

INADEQUATE RESPONSE. This may be because the wrong vitamin has been given, because the patient has an associated cause for anaemia (e.g. iron deficiency, infection or malignancy), or because the diagnosis is incorrect.

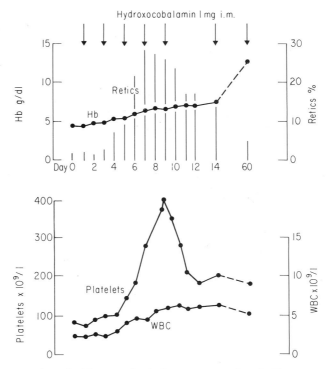

Fig. 3.10 A typical haematological response to vitamin B_{12} (hydroxocobalamin) therapy in pernicious anaemia.

OTHER MEGALOBLASTIC ANAEMIAS
(see Table 3.1)

Abnormalities of vitamin B_{12} and folate metabolism

These are unusual and include congenital deficiencies of enzymes concerned in B_{12} or folate metabolism or of the serum transport protein for B_{12}, TC II, which is needed for serum B_{12} to enter bone marrow cells. Nitrous oxide (N_2O) anaesthesia causes rapid inactivation of body vitamin B_{12} by oxidising the reduced cobalt atom of methyl B_{12}. Megaloblastic marrow changes occur within several days and prolonged N_2O administration can cause a pancytopenia. Chronic exposure (as in dentists and anaesthetists) has been associated with neurological damage resembling vitamin B_{12} deficiency neuropathy. Antifolate drugs, particularly those which inhibit dihydrofolate reductase (e.g. methotrexate and pyrimethamine) may also cause megaloblastic change (*see* p. 49). Trimethoprim, which inhibits bacterial dihydrofolate reductase, has only a slight action against the human enzyme and causes megaloblastic change only in patients already B_{12}- or folate-deficient.

Defects of DNA synthesis not related to B_{12} or folate

Congenital deficiency of one or other enzyme concerned in purine or pyrimidine synthesis may cause megaloblastic anaemia identical in appearance to that due to deficiency of vitamin B_{12} or folate. The best known is orotic aciduria. Therapy with drugs which inhibit purine or pyrimidine synthesis (such as hydroxyurea, cytosine arabinoside, and 6-mercaptopurine) also causes megaloblastic anaemia. Megaloblastic changes may also occur in association with erythroleukaemia and acquired sideroblastic anaemia but the site of the defect in DNA synthesis in these conditions is unknown and the anaemia does not respond to B_{12} or folate therapy.

CAUSES OF MACROCYTOSIS OTHER THAN MEGALOBLASTIC ANAEMIA

Big circulating red cells can be caused by a variety of conditions other than B_{12} or folate deficiency. In some of these situations the bone marrow shows normoblastic rather than megaloblastic erythropoiesis (Table 3.10). The exact mechanisms for the large red cells in each of these conditions is not clear although, in some, increased

Table 3.10 Causes of macrocytosis other than megaloblastic anaemia.

1	Alcohol
2	Liver disease
3	Myxoedema (Hypothyroidism).
4	Reticulocytosis
5	Cytotoxic drugs
6	Aplastic anaemia
7	Pregnancy , Newborn
8	Primary acquired sideroblastic anaemia and myelodysplastic syndromes
9	Myeloma
10	Respiratory failure (hypoxia) N_2O Anaesthesia (B_{12}) . →Megaloblastic A's

(handwritten annotations: "Physiological" bracketing items 6 and 7; N₂O Anaesthesia note beside item 10)

lipid deposition on the red cell membrane and, in others, alterations in blast maturation time in the marrow have been suggested. Reticulocytes are bigger than mature red cells. The red cells in the macrocytic but normoblastic anaemias usually are round rather than oval and the neutrophils are not hypersegmented. Alcohol is the most frequent cause of a raised MCV in the absence of anaemia. In some severe alcoholics, however, megaloblastic anaemia is due to a direct toxic action of alcohol on the marrow or to associated dietary deficiency of folate. The other underlying conditions listed in Table 3.10 are usually easily diagnosed provided that they are considered and the appropriate investigations to exclude B_{12} or folate deficiency (e.g. serum B_{12} and folate assay and bone marrow examination) are carried out.

Differential diagnosis of a macrocytic anaemia

The clinical history and physical examination may suggest B_{12} or folate deficiency as the cause. Diet and drugs, alcohol intake, family history, history suggestive of malabsorption, presence of auto-immune diseases, previous gastrointestinal disease or operation, are all important. The presence of jaundice, glossitis or a neuropathy are also valuable pointers to megaloblastic anaemia.

The laboratory features of particular importance are the shape of macrocytes, (oval in megaloblastic anaemia) the presence of hypersegmented neutrophils and of leucopenia and thrombocytopenia and the bone marrow appearance. Serum B_{12}, serum and red cell folate, and special tests for causes of these deficiencies are used to complete the diagnosis of megaloblastic anaemia. Exclusion of alcoholism, liver and thyroid function tests and bone marrow examination are important in the investigation of macrocytic anaemia not due to B_{12} or folate deficiency.

SELECTED BIBLIOGRAPHY

Carmel R. (1983) Megaloblastic anemia: vitamin B_{12} and folate. In
   Current Hematology, vol. 2, pp. 243–80, ed. V.F. Fairbanks. John
   Wiley, New York.
Chanarin I. (1979) *The Megaloblastic Anaemias*, 2nd edition. Blackwell
   Scientific Publications, Oxford.
Chanarin I. (1982) The effects of nitrous oxide on cobalamins, folates and
   on related events. CRC Critical Reviews on Toxicology, pp. 179–213.
   CRC Press, Florida.
Clinics in Haematology (1976) vol. 5.3. Ed. A.V. Hoffbrand. W.B.
   Saunders, Philadelphia.
Hoffbrand A.V. (1983) Pernicious Anaemia. *Scottish Medical Journal* **28**,
   218–27.
Hoffbrand A.V. & Wickremsinghe R.G. (1981) Megaloblastic anaemia.
   In *Recent Advances in Haematology* 3, pp. 95–144, ed. A.V.
   Hoffbrand. Churchill Livingstone, Edinburgh.
Kass L. (1976) Pernicious Anemia. In *Major Problems in Internal
   Medicine*, vol. 7. W.B. Saunders, Philadelphia.

Chapter 4
Haemolytic anaemia

Haemolytic anaemias are defined as those anaemias which result from an <u>increase in the rate of red cell destruction.</u> Because of erythropoietic hyperplasia and anatomical extension of bone marrow, red cell destruction may be increased several-fold before the patient becomes anaemic (compensated haemolytic disease). The adult <u>marrow, after full expansion,</u> is able to <u>produce red cells at 6–8 times the normal rate.</u> <u>Reticulocytes are raised,</u> particularly in the more anaemic cases and those in which erythropoiesis is effective (as in hereditary spherocytosis) compared to those haemolytic anaemias in which red cell production is largely ineffective (as in beta-thalassaemia major). The reticulocytes appear as larger, slightly blue-staining (polychromatic) cells in the ordinary peripheral blood film but are counted accurately after supravital staining (Fig. 1.17b).

The lifespan of the normal red cell is 120 days; in severe

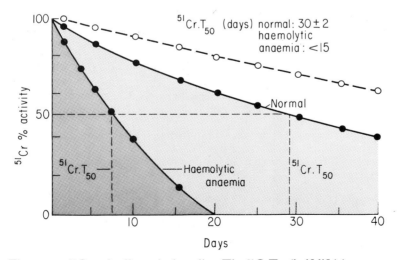

Fig. 4.1a ^{51}Cr red cell survival studies. The ^{51}CrT$_{50}$ (half-life) in normal subjects is 30 ± 2 days. When data are corrected for elution of ^{51}Cr from red cells (dotted line), the mean cell life is 50 ± 5 days. In haemolytic anaemia, the ^{51}CrT$_{50}$ is usually less than 15 days.

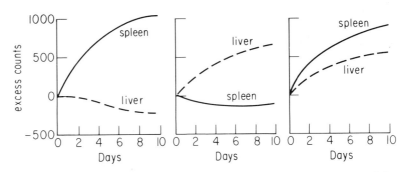

Fig. 4.1b Surface counting patterns in haemolytic anaemia during ^{51}Cr red cell survival studies. (*Left*) Dominant splenic destruction, e.g. hereditary spherocytosis. (*Centre*) Dominant liver destruction, e.g. sickle cell disease. (*Right*) Combined pattern of destruction, e.g. some cases of auto-immune haemolytic anaemia.

haemolysis the cells survive only a few days. Chromium-51 (^{51}Cr)-labelled red cell survival studies may be needed to confirm haemolysis and to determine sites of destruction by surface counting over the different organs (Fig. 4.1). Diagnosis of the type of anaemia in any particular case requires a full clinical history, including family history and drug history as well as clinical examination and appropriate laboratory tests.

Table 4.1 is a simplified classification of the haemolytic anaemias. Hereditary haemolytic anaemias are usually the result of 'intrinsic' red cell defects; normal transfused blood survives as

Table 4.1 Classification of haemolytic anaemia.

	Defect of	Disease
Hereditary	Membrane	e.g. Hereditary spherocytosis, hereditary elliptocytosis
	Metabolism	e.g. G6PD deficiency, pyruvate kinase deficiency
	Haemoglobin	1. Abnormal (Hb S, Hb C, unstable, etc.) 2. Defective synthesis (thalassaemias)
Acquired	Immune	
	Autoimmune haemolytic anaemias	
	Isoimmune, e.g. haemolytic transfusion reaction and haemolytic disease of the newborn (Chapter 14)	
	Drug-induced immune haemolytic anaemia	
	Red cell fragmentation syndromes	
	Hypersplenism	
	Secondary, e.g. renal disease, liver disease	
	Paroxysmal nocturnal haemoglobinuria	
	Miscellaneous, e.g. infections, chemicals, toxins and drugs	

long in these patients as in healthy recipients. Acquired haemolytic anaemias are usually the result of an 'extracorpuscular' or 'environmental' change; normal transfused blood will have the same short survival as the patient's own red cells in these patients.

General features of haemolysis

CLINICAL. The patient may show pallor of the mucous membranes, mild fluctuating jaundice and splenomegaly. There is no bile in the urine but this may turn dark on standing because of excess urobilinogen. Pigment gallstones may complicate the condition (Fig. 4.2) and some patients (particularly with sickle cell disease) develop ulcers around the ankle. Aplastic crises may occur, usually precipitated by infection with parvovirus which 'switches off' erythropoiesis, and are characterised by a sudden increase in anaemia and drop in reticulocyte count.

Folate deficiency is also likely to occur in chronic haemolytic anaemias because of increased utilisation of the vitamin by the rapidly proliferating (DNA synthesising) bone marrow. If severe, this may cause an aplastic crisis in which the bone marrow is megaloblastic.

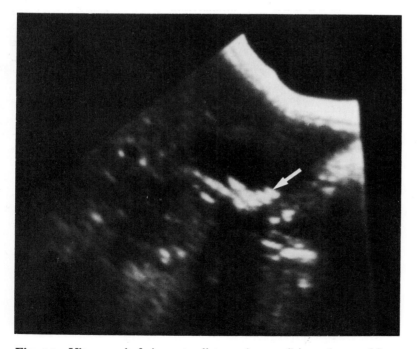

Fig. 4.2 Ultrasound of pigment gallstones (arrowed) in a 16-year-old male patient with hereditary spherocytosis. (Photograph courtesy of L. Berger.)

LABORATORY. The laboratory findings are conveniently divided into three groups:

1 *Features of increased red cell breakdown.*

Extravascular (i) Serum bilirubin raised; unconjugated; bound to albumin.

    (ii) Urine urinobilinogen — increased.

    (iii) Faecal stercobilinogen — increased.

    (iv) Serum haptoglobins (haemoglobin binding protein) — absent because the haemoglobin–haptoglobin complex is removed by RE cells.

2 *Features of increased red cell production.*

    (i) Reticulocytosis.

    (ii) Bone marrow erythroid hyperplasia.

3 *Damaged red cells.*

    (i) Morphology — microspherocytes; fragments, etc.

    (ii) Osmotic fragility, autohaemolysis, etc.

    (iii) Red cell survival shortened. Best shown by ^{51}Cr labelling with study of sites of destruction (see Fig. 4.1a & b).

PARTICULAR FEATURES OF
INTRAVASCULAR HAEMOLYSIS

In some situations the red cells may be destroyed directly in the circulation, e.g. ABO mismatched transfusion, glucose 6-phosphate dehydrogenase deficiency, some cold antibody haemolytic syndromes, some mechanical, drug and infection-induced haemolytic anaemias, paroxysmal nocturnal haemoglobinuria. The free haemoglobin released rapidly saturates plasma haptoglobins, the haemoglobin–haptoglobin complex being removed by the RE cells. The excess free haemoglobin is filtered by the glomerulus, rapidly saturates the renal tubular re-absorptive capacity and enters urine. Some of the free plasma haemoglobin is removed by hepatic macrophages and some of the haem released from this is oxidised to the trivalent iron form, released from the cell and binds to plasma albumin—forming methaemalbumin. Haem is also bound in plasma to another protein, haemopexin, which is then mainly removed by the liver.

The main laboratory features of this intravascular haemolysis are:

(i) haemoglobinaemia and haemoglobinuria;

(ii) haemosiderinuria (iron storage protein in spun deposit of urine derived from breakdown of haemoglobin being reabsorbed in renal tubular cells);

(iii) methaemalbuminaemia (detected spectrophotometrically by Schumm's test).

HEREDITARY HAEMOLYTIC ANAEMIAS

Membrane defects

HEREDITARY SPHEROCYTOSIS

This is the commonest hereditary haemolytic anaemia in north Europeans, probably due to one or other of a variety of defects in a structural protein (spectrin) of the red cell membrane. The marrow produces red cells of normal biconcave shape but these lose membrane as they circulate through the spleen and the rest of the RE system. The ratio of surface area to volume decreases and the cells become more spherical and ultimately are unable to pass through the splenic microcirculation where the spherocytes die prematurely. The reason for loss of membrane in the RE system is not certain. *In vitro*, glucose helps to prevent undue loss of sodium from the cells through the leaky membrane; and glucose deprivation has been postulated to occur particularly when the cells circulate to the spleen, perhaps because of stasis and plasma skimming.

INHERITANCE. Dominant, variable expression. *incomplete penetrance*

CLINICAL FEATURES. The anaemia may present at any age from infancy to old age. Jaundice is typically fluctuating and is particularly marked if the haemolytic anaemia is associated with Gilbert's disease (a defect of hepatic conjugation of bilirubin); *transport into Hepatocyte* splenomegaly occurs in most patients. Pigment gallstones are frequent (Fig. 4.2); 'aplastic crises' (usually precipitated by infection, nearly always parvovirus) may cause a sudden increase in severity of anaemia.

HAEMATOLOGICAL FINDINGS. Anaemia is usual but not invariable; its severity tends to be similar in members of the same family. Reticulocytes are usually 5–20%. The blood film shows microspherocytes (Fig. 4.3a) which are densely staining with smaller diameters than normal red cells, particularly reticulocytes.

SPECIAL TESTS

1 *Osmotic fragility is increased* (Fig. 4.3b). The abnormality may require 24 hours' incubation at 37°C to become obvious.
2 *Autohaemolysis is increased* and corrected by glucose. In this test, the cells are incubated in their own plasma for 48 hours and the degree of haemolysis is measured.
3 *Direct Coombs' (antiglobulin) test is negative.* This excludes auto-immune haemolysis in which spherocytes are also common.
4 *^{51}Cr studies* are used to assess the severity and document dominant splenic destruction (Figs. 4.1a and 4.1b).

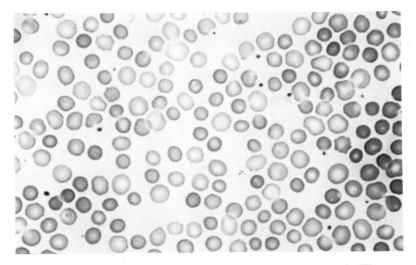

Fig. 4.3a The peripheral blood film in hereditary spherocytosis. The spherocytes are densely staining and of small diameter.

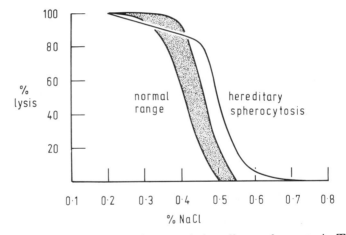

Fig. 4.3b The osmotic fragility curve in hereditary spherocytosis. The curve is shifted to the right of the (shaded) normal range, but a tail of more resistant cells (reticulocytes) is also present.

TREATMENT

Splenectomy. This is avoided in early childhood, if possible, because of the increased risk of infection (particularly pneumococcal) post-splenectomy at this age. Splenectomy should always produce a rise in the haemoglobin level to normal, even though microspherocytes (formed in the rest of the RE system) remain. Folic acid is given in severe cases and pneumococcal vaccination is also given before splenectomy is undertaken.

This has similar clinical and laboratory features to hereditary spherocytosis except for the appearance of the blood film, but it is usually a clinically milder disorder. Occasional patients require splenectomy. Defective spectrin dimer-dimer association in the red cell membrane or a deficit in interaction of spectrin with other membrane proteins have been detected in different cases.

Defective red cell metabolism

GLUCOSE 6-PHOSPHATE DEHYDROGENASE (G6PD) DEFICIENCY

There are a wide variety of normal genetic variants of the enzyme G6PD, the commonest being type B (Western) and type A in Negroes. Numerous variants of the enzyme G6PD have been characterised which show less activity than normal. These abnormalities are due to a deficiency of the enzyme protein or to a functional inadequacy of the enzyme. There is impaired reduction of glutathione (Fig. 4.4). The main syndrome which occurs is acute haemolytic anaemia in response to oxidant stress (drugs, fava beans) but neonatal jaundice, haemolysis due to infections, and, rarely, a congenital non-spherocytic haemolytic anaemia result from different types of enzyme deficiency.

The inheritance is sex-linked, affecting males, and carried by females who show approximately half normal red cell G6PD

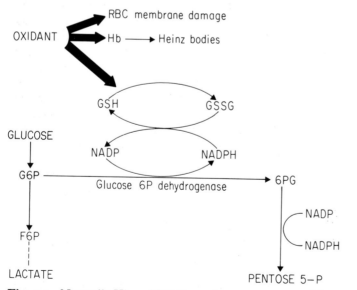

Fig. 4.4 Normally Hb and R B C membrane are protected from oxidant stress by reduced glutathione (GSH). In G6PD deficiency, NADPH and GSH synthesis is impaired. (*See* Fig. 1.14 for abbreviations.)

values. The main races affected are in West Africa, the Mediterranean, the Middle East and South-East Asia. The degree of deficiency varies, often being mild (10–15% of normal activity) in Negroes, more severe in Orientals and most severe in Mediterraneans. Severe deficiency occurs occasionally in Caucasians.

CLINICAL FEATURES. These are of rapid developing intravascular haemolysis precipitated by infection and other acute illness, drugs or the ingestion of the fava bean (Table 4.2). In Negroes the anaemia is self-limiting because the new young red cells have near normal G6PD activity, the enzyme level falling as the cells age in the circulation. In contrast, in the Mediterranean type of deficiency, haemolysis is not necessarily self-limiting.

Table 4.2   Agents which may cause haemolytic anaemia in G6PD deficiency.

1	*Infections and other acute illnesses, e.g. diabetic ketoacidosis*
2	*Drugs:*
	a anti-malarials, e.g. primaquine, pyrimethamine, quinine, chloroquine
	b analgesics, e.g. phenacetin, acetylsalicylic acid, paracetamol
	c anti-bacterial, e.g. sulphonamides, nitrofurones, penicillin, isoniazid, streptomycin
	d miscellaneous, e.g. vitamin K, probenecid, quinidine, dapsone
3	*Fava beans* (possibly other vegetables)

DIAGNOSIS. Between crises the blood count is normal. The enzyme deficiency is detected by one of a number of screening tests or by direct enzyme assay on red cells. During a crisis, the blood film may show contracted and fragmented cells, 'bite' cells and 'blister' cells which have had Heinz bodies removed by the spleen (Fig. 4.5). Heinz bodies (oxidised, denatured haemoglobin) may be seen in the reticulocyte preparation, particularly if the spleen is absent (Fig. 1.17b). There are also features of intravascular haemolysis (see p. 62). Because of the higher enzyme level in young red cells, red cell enzyme assay may give a 'false' normal level in the phase of acute haemolysis with a reticulocyte response. Subsequent assay after the acute phase reveals the low G6PD level when the red cell population is of normal age distribution.

TREATMENT. The offending drug is stopped, a high urine output is maintained, and blood transfusion undertaken where necessary for severe anaemia.

Other defects in the pentose phosphate pathway leading to similar syndromes to G6PD deficiency have been described—particularly glutathione deficiency.

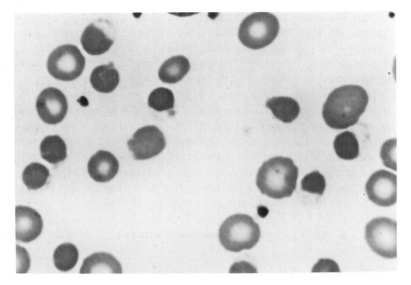

Fig. 4.5 Peripheral blood in a patient with glucose 6-phosphate dehydrogenase deficiency and acute haemolysis after ingestion of fava beans. Some of the red cells show loss of cytoplasm with separation of remaining haemoglobin away from the cell membrane ('blister' cells). There are also numerous contracted and densely staining red cells. The haemolysis is largely intravascular. Supravital staining (as for reticulocytes) shows the presence of Heinz bodies (see Fig. 1.17b).

Glycolytic (Embden–Meyerhof) pathway defects

These are all uncommon and lead to a congenital non-spherocytic haemolytic anaemia. The most frequently encountered is pyruvate kinase deficiency.

PYRUVATE KINASE (PK) DEFICIENCY. This is inherited as an autosomal recessive, the affected patients being homozygous. The red cells become rigid due to reduced ATP formation. The anaemia (haemoglobin 4–10 g/dl) causes relatively mild symptoms because of a shift to the right in the O_2-dissociation curve because of a rise in intracellular 2,3-DPG. The blood film shows poikilocytosis and distorted cells. Laboratory tests show that autohaemolysis is increased but, in contrast to hereditary spherocytosis, it is not corrected by glucose; direct enzyme assay is needed to make the diagnosis. The enzyme often shows abnormal characteristics as well as reduced activity. Splenectomy may alleviate the anaemia but does not cure it.

Haemoglobin abnormalities

Normal foetal and adult haemoglobin synthesis is discussed on p. 8. Hereditary haemoglobin abnormalities are divided into two main groups:

1 *Synthesis of an abnormal haemoglobin.* These contain an amino acid substitution in either the α or β globin chain. A variety of different syndromes may occur depending on the type and site of substitution (Table 4.3); in many the abnormality is completely silent. By far the most important of these diseases is sickle cell anaemia. Haemoglobins C, D and E are also common (Fig. 4.5) and, in the homozygous states, produce a mild haemolytic anaemia for which no treatment is needed. The rare unstable haemoglobins cause chronic haemolysis of varying severity. There are Heinz bodies in the peripheral blood and the haemoglobin is heat labile. Abnormal haemoglobins can also cause other clinical syndromes, e.g. polycythaemia (p. 184) or one variety of congenital methaemoglobinaemia (Table 4.3).

2 *Reduced synthesis of normal globin chains.* This includes the alpha- and beta-thalassaemias in which synthesis of one or other globin chain is reduced.

Table 4.3 The clinical syndromes produced by structural haemoglobin abnormalities (single amino acid substitutions in the α or β chain).

Insoluble haemoglobin
1 Crystalline haemoglobin★
  (Hb S, C, D, E, etc.) $\Big\} \rightarrow$ haemolysis
2 Unstable haemoglobin

Abnormal oxygen transport
1 Altered affinity $\rightarrow$ polycythaemia
2 Failure of reduction (Hb M's) $\rightarrow$ methaemoglobinaemia (cyanosis)

★ These are the only common disorders in this group

GEOGRAPHICAL DISTRIBUTION

Fig. 4.6 shows the main areas where these haemoglobin disorders occur. Sickle cell trait affords protection against *P. falciparum* malaria which may explain its persistence in tropical and subtropical areas; however, the explanation for the distribution of the other disorders is unclear.

Sickle cell anaemia

Hb S (Hb $\alpha_2\beta^S{}_2$) is insoluble and forms crystals when exposed to low oxygen tension, the red cells sickle and may block different areas of the microcirculation causing infarcts of various organs. The abnormality is due to substitution of valine for glutamic acid in position 6 in the β chain (Fig. 4.7).

HOMOZYGOUS DISEASE

CLINICAL FEATURES. These are of a severe haemolytic anaemia punctuated by *crises*. The symptoms of anaemia are often mild

Haemolytic anaemia   69

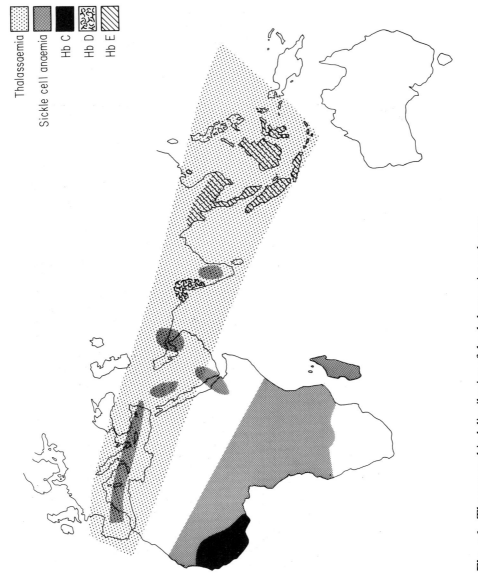

Fig. 4.6 The geographical distribution of the thalassaemias and more common inherited structural haemoglobin abnormalities.

Normal β chain	amino acid	pro	glu	glu
	base composition	CCT	G͡AG	GAG
Sickle β chain	base composition	CCT	G͜TG	GAG
	amino acid	pro	val	glu

Fig. 4.7 Molecular pathology of sickle cell anaemia. There is a single base change in the DNA coding for the amino-acid in the sixth position in the β globin chain (adenine is replaced by thymine). This leads to an aminoacid change from glutamic acid to valine.
pro = proline, glu = glutamic acid, val = valine, C = cytosine, T = thymine, A = adenine, G = guanine.

in relation to the severity of the anaemia since Hb S gives up oxygen to tissues relatively easily compared with Hb A. Crises may be painful, aplastic, haemolytic or infectious. Painful crises are precipitated by such factors as infection, dehydration or deoxygenation (e.g. altitude, operations, obstetric delivery, stasis of the circulation, exposure to cold, violent exercise, etc.). Infarcts may occur in a variety of organs including bones, the lungs, and the spleen. In children, the 'hand-foot' syndrome of painful dactylitis due to infarcts of the small bones is frequent and may lead to digits of varying lengths (Fig. 4.8). Osteomyelitis, sometimes due to salmonella may develop in infarcted bones. Haematuria and failure of urine concentration may occur due to renal infarcts. 'Aplastic' crises may also occur due to infection with parvovirus and/or folate deficiency and are characterised by a sudden fall in haemo-

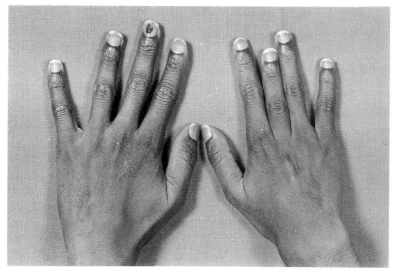

Fig. 4.8a The hands in a 22-year-old Nigerian man with homozygous sickle cell disease. There is shortening of the right middle finger.

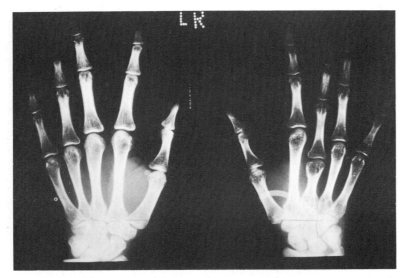

Fig. 4.8b X-ray of hands of patient in Fig. 4.8a. There is shortening of the third right metacarpal. This is due to infarction of the metaphysis in childhood. There were similar abnormalities in the toes of both feet ('hand-foot' syndrome). Tubing for intravenous rehydration during a crisis is also apparent.

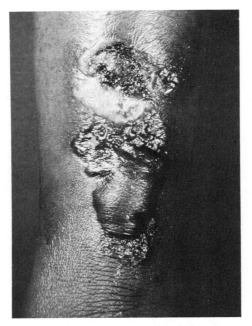

Fig. 4.8c Ulceration above the ankle in a 16-year-old patient with homozygous sickle cell anaemia.

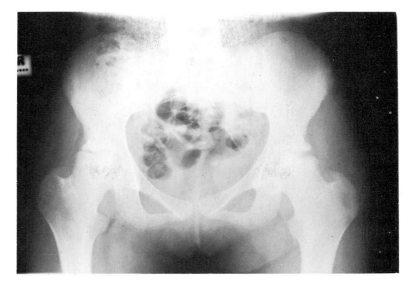

Fig. 4.9 X-ray of hip joints of a young adult patient with homozygous sickle cell disease. There is severe joint damage due to bone infarcts.

↓Hbglobin concentration and fall in reticulocyte count. Ulcers of the lower legs are common, due to vascular stasis and local ischaemia (Fig. 4.8c). The spleen is enlarged in infancy and early childhood but later is often reduced in size due to infarcts (autosplenectomy).

LABORATORY DIAGNOSIS
(i) The haemoglobin is usually 6–9 g/dl—low in comparison to symptoms of anaemia.
(ii) Sickle cells and target cells occur in the blood (Fig. 4.10). Features of splenic atrophy (e.g. Howell–Jolly bodies, Fig. 1.17b) may also be present.
(iii) Screening tests for sickling when the blood is deoxygenated with dithionate and Na_2HPO_4.
(iv) Haemoglobin electrophoresis (Fig. 4.14). In Hb SS, no normal Hb A is detected. The amount of Hb F is variable and is usually 5–15%; larger amounts are normally associated with a milder disorder, e.g. so-called benign sickle cell anaemia in the Middle East.

TREATMENT
(i) Prophylactic—avoid those factors known to precipitate crises (see above).
(ii) Folic acid, e.g. 5 mg daily, if the diet is poor.
(iii) Good general nutrition and hygiene.
(iv) Crisis—rest, rehydrate, give antibiotics if infection is present, bicarbonate if the patient is acidotic. Strong analgesics are usually

Haemolytic anaemia   73

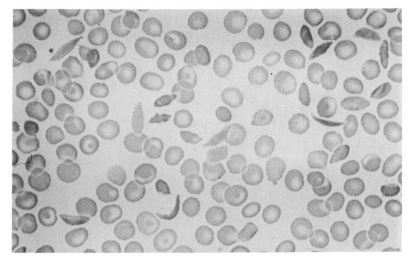

Fig. 4.10 The peripheral blood in sickle cell anaemia. Note the deeply staining sickle cells and target cells.

needed. Transfusion is given only if there is very severe anaemia with symptoms. Exchange transfusion may be needed in severe cases.

(v) Particular care is needed in pregnancy and anaesthesia. Before delivery or operations, patients may be transfused repeatedly with normal blood to reduce the proportion of circulating haemoglobin S.

(vi) Transfusions—these are also sometimes given to patients having frequent crises to suppress Hb S production completely over a period of several months.

SICKLE CELL TRAIT. This is a benign condition with no anaemia and normal appearance of red cells but crises can occur with extreme stress, e.g. anoxia and severe infections. Haematuria may occur. Haemoglobin S varies from 25 to 45% of the total. Care must be taken with anaesthesia and in pregnancy.

COMBINATION OF HB S WITH OTHER
HAEMOGLOBINOPATHIES

The commonest are S-thalassaemia and S-C disease, which behave like mild forms of sickle cell disease. Patients with S-C disease have a particular tendency to thrombosis and pulmonary embolism, especially in pregnancy. Diagnosis is made by haemoglobin electrophoresis, particularly with family studies.

HAEMOGLOBIN C DISEASE. This is frequent in West Africa and is due to substitution of lysine for glutamic acid in the β chain at the same point as the substitution in Hb S. Hb C tends to form rhomboidal crystals and in the homozygous state there is a mild haemolytic anaemia with marked target cell formation and micro spherocytes; the spleen is enlarged.

Thalassaemias

α-THALASSAEMIA SYNDROMES

These are listed in Table 4.4. As there is duplication of the α globin chain gene, deletion of 4 genes is needed to completely suppress α chain synthesis. Since the α chain is needed in foetal as well as in adult haemoglobin, α^4 gene deletion leads to failure of foetal haemoglobin synthesis with death *in utero* (hydrops foetalis). Three gene deletion leads to a moderately severe (haemoglobin 7–11 g/dl) microcytic, hypochromic anaemia with splenomegaly (haemoglobin H disease) in which haemoglobin H (β^4) can be detected in red cells by electrophoresis or in reticulocyte preparations. In foetal life, haemoglobin Bart's (γ^4) occurs.

The α-thalassaemia traits are often not associated with anaemia, but the MCV, MCH and MCHC are all low and the red cell count is over $5.5 \times 10^{12}/l$. Haemoglobin electrophoresis is normal but occasionally haemoglobin H bodies may be observed in isolated red cells in reticulocyte preparations and α/β chain synthesis ratio studies are needed to be certain of the diagnosis. The normal α/β ratio is 1:1 and it is reduced in the α-thalassaemias. Uncommon forms of α-thalassaemia are due to genetic lesions other than gene deletions.

Table 4.4 The thalassaemias.

Genetic abnormality	Clinical syndrome
α-thalassaemias	
4 gene deletion—hydrops foetalis	lethal *in utero*
3 gene deletion—haemoglobin H disease	haemolytic anaemia
2 gene deletion (α° thalassaemia trait)	microcytic, hypochromic, blood
1 gene deletion (α⁺ thalassaemia trait)	picture but usually no anaemia
β-thalassaemias	
homozygous—β-thalassaemia major	severe anaemia requires blood transfusions
heterozygous—thalassaemia trait	blood film hypochromic and microcytic; anaemia mild or absent
Thalassaemia intermedia a clinical syndrome due to a variety of genetic lesions (*see* p. 79)	hypochromic, microcytic anaemia (Hb 7.0–10.0 g/dl); enlarged liver and spleen, bone deformities, iron overload

β-Thalassaemia syndromes—β-thalassaemia major

This condition is also known as Mediterranean or Cooley's anaemia and occurs in 1 in 4 offspring if two carriers of β-thalassaemia trait marry. Either no β chain (β^0) or small amounts (β^+) are synthesised. Excess α chains precipitate in erythroblasts and mature red cells causing <u>severe ineffective erythropoiesis</u> and <u>haemolysis</u>. Over 20 different genetic defects have now been detected, some being particularly common in certain racial groups (Table 4.5).

Table 4.5 Some of the more common genetic lesions responsible for β-thalassaemia. (Courtesy D.J. Weatherall.)

Nonsense mutations	β^0	⎫
Splice junction mutations	β^0	⎬ Mediterranean
Cryptic splice sites	β^+	⎱ Oriental
Frame shifts	β^0	⎭
Partial deletion	β^0	N. India
Promotor site mutations	β^+	Mediterranean

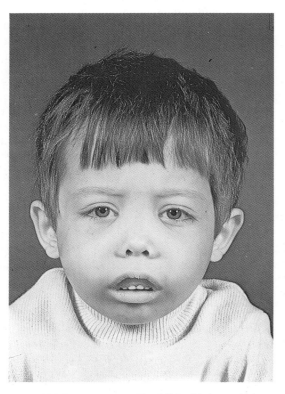

Fig. 4.11 The facial appearance of a child with beta-thalassaemia major. The skull is bossed with prominent frontal and parietal bones, the maxilla is enlarged.

CLINICAL FEATURES

(i) Severe anaemia becomes apparent at 3–6 months after birth when the switch from γ to β chain production should take place.
(ii) Enlargement of the liver and spleen occurs due to excessive red cell destruction, extramedullary haemopoiesis and iron overload. The large spleen increases blood requirements by increasing red cell destruction and pooling and by causing expansion of the plasma volume.
(iii) Expansion of bones due to intense marrow hyperplasia leads to a thalassaemic facies (Fig. 4.11), thinning of cortex of many bones with a tendency to fractures and hair-on-end appearance of the skull on X-ray (Fig. 4.12).

Iron overload due to repeated transfusions (each 500 ml transfused contains about 250 mg iron) causes damage to the liver, the endocrine organs (with failure of growth, delayed or absent puberty, diabetes mellitus, etc.), and to the myocardium with ultimate death in the absence of intensive iron chelation in the 2nd or 3rd decade from congestive heart failure or cardiac arrhythmias. Clinical abnormalities usually appear after 100 units (25 g iron) have been transfused. Investigation of iron overload is discussed on p. 39.

DIAGNOSIS

(i) There is a severe hypochromic microcytic anaemia with raised reticulocyte percentage with normoblasts, target cells and basophilic stippling in the blood film (Fig. 4.13).
(ii) Haemoglobin electrophoresis reveals absence or almost complete absence of Hb A with almost all the haemoglobin circulating Hb F. The Hb A_2 per cent is normal, low, or slightly raised (Fig. 4.14). α/β chain synthesis studies on circulating reticulocytes show marked increase in the α/β ratio, i.e. reduced or absent β chain synthesis.

TREATMENT

(i) Regular blood transfusions are needed to maintain Hb over 11 g/dl. This usually requires 2–3 units every 4-6 weeks. Fresh blood, filtered to remove white cells, gives the best red cell survival with the fewest reactions.
(ii) Regular folic acid (e.g. 5 mg daily), if the diet is poor.
(iii) Iron chelation therapy is used to prevent iron overload. Desferrioxamine is given, 2 g with each unit of blood transfused, and also by daily subcutaneous infusion (1-4 g over 8-12 hours). Chelated iron is largely excreted in urine as ferrioxamine and, in heavily iron-loaded cases, excretion rates of up to 200 mg of iron daily can be achieved. With this intensive iron chelation regime, the outlook for these children may have improved but long-term follow-up has not yet been carried out.

Haemolytic anaemia 77

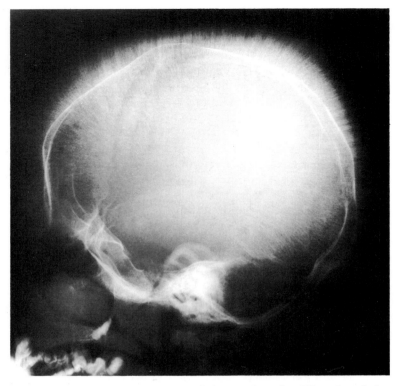

Fig. 4.12 The skull X-ray in beta-thalassaemia major. There is an hair-on-end appearance due to expansion of the bone marrow into cortical bone.

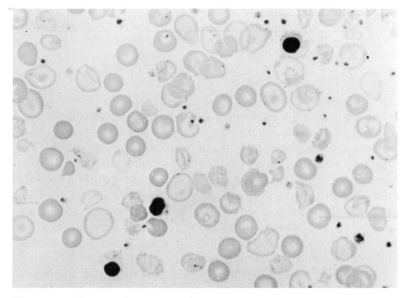

Fig. 4.13 The peripheral blood film in beta-thalassaemia major, post-splenectomy. Note the target and hypochromic cells, presence of normoblasts. Some of the mature red cells contain small granules (Pappenheimer bodies) or Howell–Jolly bodies due to splenectomy. The well haemoglobinised cells are from transfused blood.

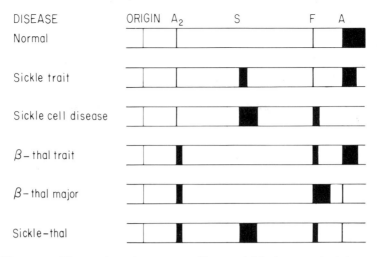

Fig. 4.14 Electrophoretic patterns of haemoglobin in normal adult human blood and in subjects with sickle cell disease or β-thalassaemia. In the last two conditions shown in the figure, haemoglobin A may be completely absent or present only in small amounts.

(iv) Vitamin C, 200 mg daily, increases excretion of iron produced by desferrioxamine.

(v) Splenectomy may be needed to reduce blood requirements. This is delayed until the patient is over 6 years old because of the risk of infection. Pneumococcal vaccine and/or prophylactic penicillin therapy are given after splenectomy.

(vi) Endocrine therapy is given either as replacement or to stimulate the pituitary if puberty is delayed.

(vii) In a few cases bone marrow transplantation has been carried out successfully in the first year or two of life from an HLA-matched sibling.

Thalassaemia intermedia

Some cases of β-thalassaemia of moderate severity (haemoglobin 7.0–10.0 g/dl) who do not need regular transfusions are called 'thalassaemia intermedia'. This is a clinical syndrome, therefore, which may be due to a variety of genetic defects. It may be due to homozygous β-thalassaemia with production of more haemoglobin F than usual, or with a mild defect in β-chain synthesis, or to β-thalassaemia trait of unusual severity alone, or in association with other mild globin abnormalities, e.g. Hb E or Hb Lepore. The coexistence of α-thalassaemia trait also improves the haemoglobin level in homozygous β-thalassaemia by reducing the degree of chain imbalance and thus of α-chain precipitation and ineffective erythropoiesis. The patient with thalassaemia intermedia shows bone deformity, enlarged liver and spleen, extramedullary erythropoiesis and features of iron overload in adulthood.

β-thalassaemia trait (minor)

A common, usually symptomless abnormality characterised by a markedly hypochromic, microcytic blood picture (MCV, MCH and MCHC all very low) but mild or no anaemia (Hb 11–15 g/dl). A raised Hb A_2 (>3.5%) confirms the diagnosis. The results of iron studies are normal. If two subjects with β-thalassaemia trait ('carriers') marry, there is a 25% chance of a thalassaemia major offspring. Antenatal diagnosis and abortion can prevent this. 50% of their offspring will be carriers.

Haemoglobin Lepore

This is an abnormal haemoglobin due to unequal crossing over of the β and δ genes to produce a polypeptide chain consisting of the δ-chain at its amino end and β-chain at its carboxyl end. The δβ fusion chain is synthesised inefficiently and normal δ and β-chain production is abolished. The homozygotes show thalassaemia intermedia and the heterozygotes show thalassaemia trait.

ANTENATAL DIAGNOSIS OF THE HAEMOGLOBINOPATHIES

Antenatal diagnosis of haemoglobinopathies may be performed either by examining globin chain synthesis in foetal blood obtained by foetoscopy or by using cDNA probes to hybridise with foetal DNA obtained either by amniocentesis or by trophoblast biopsy. The procedures carry a risk, but are indicated in order to prevent the birth of a child with β-thalassaemia major. If the parents and physicians agree, these procedures can also be used to prevent the birth of a child with other major haemoglobin defects.

ACQUIRED HAEMOLYTIC ANAEMIAS

Auto-immune haemolytic anaemias (AIHA)

These anaemias are due to antibody production by the body against its own red cells. They are characterised by a positive direct Coombs' (antiglobulin) test (see Fig. 14.1) and divided into 'warm' and 'cold' types (Table 4.6) according to whether the antibody reacts better with red cells at 37°C or 4°C.

[handwritten margin note: → Ab or complement on RBC surface?]

WARM AIHA

The red cells are usually coated with IgG either alone or with complement but a minority of cases show IgA or IgM coating alone or combined with IgG antibody. The AIHA in SLE is typically of the IgG + complement type. Red cells coated with IgG

Table 4.6 Auto-immune haemolytic anaemias: classification.

Warm type	Cold type
Idiopathic	Idiopathic
Secondary	Secondary
SLE, other 'auto-immune'	Infections — mycoplasma
diseases	pneumonia, infectious
CLL, lymphomas	mononucleosis
Drugs, e.g. methyl dopa	Lymphoma
	Paroxysmal cold haemoglobinuria
	Rare, sometimes associated with
	infections, e.g. syphilis

are taken up by RE macrophages, especially in the spleen, which have receptors for the Fc fragment. Part of the coated membrane is lost so the cell becomes progressively more spherical to maintain the same volume and is ultimately prematurely destroyed, usually predominantly in the spleen. Red cells with complement coating in addition to IgG are destroyed more generally in the RE system, and not particularly in the spleen.

CLINICAL FEATURES. The disease may occur at any age in either sex and presents as a haemolytic anaemia of varying severity. The spleen is often enlarged. The disease tends to remit and relapse. It may occur alone or in association with other diseases or arise in some patients as a result of methyl dopa therapy (Table 4.6).

LABORATORY DIAGNOSIS. The haematological and biochemical findings are typical of a haemolytic anaemia with spherocytosis prominent in the peripheral blood. The direct Coombs' (antiglobulin) test (DAT) is positive with IgG, IgG and complement, IgA (or, rarely, IgM) on the cells. In some cases, the auto-antibody shows specificity within the rhesus system, e.g. anti-c or anti-e (see Chapter 14). The antibodies both on the cell surface and free in serum are best detected at 37°C.

TREATMENT
(i) Remove the underlying cause (e.g. methyl dopa).
(ii) Corticosteroids. Prednisolone in high — subsequently reducing — doses may be tried (60 mg daily is a usual starting dose).
(iii) Splenectomy may be of value in those who fail to respond well or to maintain a satisfactory haemoglobin level on an acceptably small steroid dosage. ^{51}Cr organ uptake studies pre-operatively confirm whether or not the spleen is the dominant site of destruction (Fig. 4.1b) and thus may be used to predict the value of splenectomy. Patients with IgG only on the red cells usually respond better to steroid therapy and to splenectomy than those with IgG and complement or with IgA.

(iv) Immunosuppression may be tried after the other measures have failed but is not always of great value. Azathioprine, cyclophosphamide and chlorambucil have been tried.

(v) Folic acid is given to severe cases and blood transfusion may be needed.

COLD AIHA

In these syndromes the auto-antibody, whether monoclonal (as in the idopathic cold haemagglutinin syndrome) or polyclonal (as following infection) attaches to red cells mainly in the peripheral circulation where the blood temperature is cooled. The antibody is usually IgM and binds to red cells best at 4°C. Depending on the titre of antibody in serum, its affinity for red cells, its ability to bind complement, and its thermal amplitude (whether or not it binds to red cells at 37°C) haemolytic syndromes of varying severity may occur. Often agglutination of red cells by the antibody causes peripheral circulation abnormalities. The antibody may then detach from red cells when they pass to the warmer central circulation but, if complement has been bound, the Coombs' test remains positive — of complement-only type — and the cells are liable to be destroyed in the whole RE system, especially the liver, giving rise to a chronic haemolytic anaemia. Intravascular haemolysis occurs in some of the syndromes, in which the complement sequence is completed on the red cell surface. Low serum levels of complement in other cases may help to protect the patient from a more severe clinical disease.

In nearly all these cold AIHA syndromes, the antibody is directed against the 'I' antigen on the red cell surface or the foetal equivalent of this, the 'i' antigen.

Paroxysmal cold haemoglobinuria is a rare syndrome of acute intravascular haemolysis after exposure to the cold in those with the Donath–Landsteiner antibody, which binds to red cells in the cold but causes lysis with complement in the warm. Viral infections and syphilis are predisposing causes.

CLINICAL FEATURES. The patient may have a chronic haemolytic anaemia aggravated by the cold and often associated with intravascular haemolysis and Raynaud's phenomenon. The patient may develop problems with the peripheral circulation, e.g. tip of nose, ears, fingers and toes, due to the agglutination of red cells in small vessels. Some secondary cases are transient after an infection, particularly mycoplasma pneumonia or infectious mononucleosis (see Table 4.6).

LABORATORY FEATURES. These are similar to those of warm AIHA except spherocytosis is less marked, red cells agglutinate in the cold, e.g. on the blood film made at room temperature, and the direct Coombs' test reveals complement only (C_3) on the red cell surface. Serum antibodies often present in high titre are IgM, react best at 4°C, and usually show specificity to antigen 'I' or 'i'. In the rare cold AIHA, paroxysmal cold haemoglobinuria, the antibody is IgG and has 'P' blood group specificity.

TREATMENT. This consists of keeping the patient warm and treating the underlying cause, if present. Alkylating agents (e.g. chlorambucil) may be helpful in the chronic varieties.

Iso-immune haemolytic anaemias

In these anaemias, antibody produced by one individual reacts with red cells of another. The two important situations, transfusion of ABO incompatible blood and rhesus disease of the newborn (see Table 4.1) are considered in Chapter 14.

Drug-induced immune haemolytic anaemias

Drugs may cause immune HA by three different mechanisms (Fig. 4.15): antibody directed against a drug-red cell membrane complex (e.g. penicillin or cephalothin), deposition of complement via drug-protein (antigen) -antibody complex on the red cells (e.g.

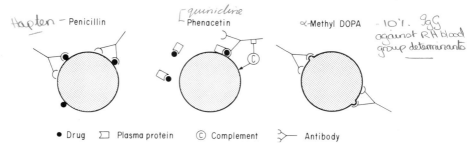

Hapten – Penicillin   [quinidine / Phenacetin   α-Methyl DOPA – 10'/. IgG against RH blood group determinants

• Drug   ⊐ Plasma protein   © Complement   >— Antibody

Fig. 4.15 Three different mechanisms of drug-induced immune haemolytic anaemia. In each case the coated (opsonized) cells are destroyed in the RE system.

phenacetin, quinidine or chlorpropamide), or an auto-immune haemolytic anaemia in which the role of the drug is mysterious (e.g. α-methyl dopa). In each case, the haemolytic anaemia gradually disappears when the drug is discontinued but with methyl dopa the auto-antibody may persist for several months. The penicillin-induced immune haemolytic anaemias only occur with massive doses of the antibiotic.

Red cell fragmentation syndromes

These arise through physical damage to red cells either on abnormal surfaces (e.g. artificial heart valves or arterial grafts) or in passing through fibrin strands deposited in small vessels due to <u>disseminated intravascular coagulation (DIC)</u> when a *micro-angiopathic haemolytic anaemia* results, e.g. in Gram-negative septicaemia, <u>malignant hypertension</u>, the <u>haemolytic-uraemic syndrome</u>, <u>mucin-secreting adenocarcinomas or thrombotic thrombocytopenic purpura</u>. The peripheral blood contains many deeply staining red cell fragments (Fig. 4.16). Clotting abnormalities typical of DIC (see p. 233) with a low platelet count are also present when DIC underlies the haemolysis. *March haemoglobinuria* is due to damage to red cells between the <u>small bones of the feet</u>, <u>usually during prolonged marching or running</u>.

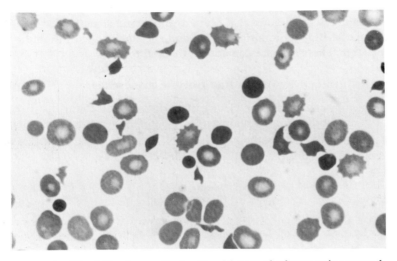

Fig. 4.16 Blood film in a patient with widespread adenocarcinoma and haemolytic anaemia due to red cell fragmentation. There are many deeply stained, fragmented, distorted, crenated and spherocytic red cells. Platelets are scanty.

Hypersplenism

Anaemia is common in patients with massive splenomegaly from any cause. Contributing factors include <u>splenic red cell pooling</u>, the dilutional element of the associated <u>increase in plasma volume</u> and a moderate haemolytic component. There is usually <u>neutropenia and thrombocytopenia</u> and the relative severity of the three cytopenias depends on the nature of the underlying disease. Frequent causes of hypersplenism include <u>portal hypertension</u>, <u>rheumatoid arthritis</u> (Felty's syndrome), <u>infections</u> (e.g. malaria, kala azar), <u>lymphomas, sarcoid, Gaucher's disease</u>, and lipid storage diseases (e.g. Niemann-Pick disease). Splenectomy or a reduction in splenic size by appropriate therapy relieves the anaemia and improves the neutrophil and platelet counts.

Secondary

In many systemic disorders red cell survival is shortened. This may contribute to anaemia (see p. 39). In renal failure, a bizarre blood film is seen with 'burr' cells, while in liver disease acanthocytes and target cells are prominent (Chapters 1 and 5).

Paroxysmal nocturnal haemoglobinuria (PNH)

This is a rare acquired defect of the red cell membrane which renders it sensitive to lysis by complement causing chronic intravascular haemolysis. It sometimes occurs in association with aplastic anaemia, especially in the recovery phase. The white cell and platelet counts are also often low in PNH because these cells share the red cells' undue sensitivity to complement. As well as the problem of anaemia, the patient may develop recurrent venous thromboses. PNH is diagnosed by demonstration of red cell lysis at low pH (acid lysis or Ham test). Haemosiderinuria is a feature and the reticulocyte count is lower in relation to the degree of anaemia than in other chronic haemolytic anaemias.

Treatment is unsatisfactory. Iron therapy is used for iron deficiency. In time, the disease occasionally remits or may transform into aplastic anaemia or acute leukaemia.

Miscellaneous haemolytic anaemias

Malaria is an important cause of haemolysis. Other infections producing haemolysis include clostridia and bartonella. Haemolytic anaemias may be caused by extensive burns, overdose with oxidising drugs (e.g. dapsone or phenacetin), chemical poisoning (e.g. lead, chlorate or arsine) and snake and spider bites. Hypophosphataemia (e.g. during intravenous feeding) leads to haemolysis due to impaired glycolysis.

SELECTED BIBLIOGRAPHY

Beutler E. (1978) *Hemolytic Anemia in Disorders of Red Cell Membrane.* Plenum Medical, New York.

Clinics in Haematology (1980) vol. 9.2, *The porphyrias.* Eds A. Goldberg & M.R. Moore. W.B. Saunders, Philadelphia.

Clinics in Haematology (1981) vol. 10.1, *Enzymopathies.* Ed. W.C. Mentzer. W.B. Saunders, Philadelphia.

Dacie J.V. (1967-1981) *The Haemolytic Anaemias,* vols 1-4. Churchill Livingstone, Edinburgh.

Fleming A.F. (ed.) (1982) *Sickle-cell Disease.* Churchill-Livingstone, Edinburgh.

Grimes A.J. (1980) *Human Red Cell Metabolism.* Blackwell Scientific Publications, Oxford.

Higgs D.R. & Weatherall D.J. (1983) Alpha thalassemia. In *Current Topics in Hematology*, vol. 4, pp. 37–97, eds S. Piomelli & S. Yachnin. Alan Liss, New York.

Lehmann H. & Huntsman R.G. (1974) *Man's Haemoglobins*, 2nd edition. North Holland, Amsterdam.

Lehmann H. & Kynoch P.A.M. (1976) *Human Haemoglobin Variants and their Characteristics*. North Holland, Amsterdam.

Methods in Hematology (1983) vol. 6. *The Thalassaemias*, Ed. D.J. Weatherall. Churchill Livingstone, Edinburgh.

Orkin S.H. *et al* (1983) Polymorphism and molecular pathology of the human beta-globin gene. *Progress in Hematology, XIII*, 49–74. Ed. E.B. Brown. Grune and Stratton, New York.

Petz L.D. & Garratty G. (1980) *Acquired Immune Haemolytic Anemias*. Churchill Livingstone, Edinburgh.

Schrier S.L. (1981) The red cell membrane and its abnormalities. In *Recent Advances in Haematology 3*, ed. A.V. Hoffbrand. Churchill Livingstone, Edinburgh.

Seminars in Haematology (1979) vols I, II, & III, *Blood Cell Membranes*. Ed. H.S. Jacob. Grune and Stratton, New York.

Seminars in Hematology (1983) vol. 20, *The Blood Cell Cytoskeleton*. Ed. J. Palek. Grune and Stratton, New York.

Sergeant G. (1976) *Sickle-Cell Anaemia*. North Holland, Amsterdam.

Warth J.A. & Rucknagel D.L. (1983) The increasing complexity of sickle cell anemia. *Progress in Hematology, XIII*, 25–48. Ed. E.B. Brown. Grune and Stratton, New York.

Weatherall D.J. & Clegg J.B. (1981) *The Thalassaemia Syndromes*, 3rd edition. Blackwell Scientific Publications, Oxford.

Chapter 5
Aplastic anaemia and anaemia in systemic diseases

APLASTIC ANAEMIA

Aplastic (hypoplastic) anaemia is defined as pancytopenia (anaemia, leucopenia and thrombocytopenia) resulting from aplasia of the bone marrow. It is classified into primary types which include a congenital form (Fanconi anaemia) and an acquired form with no obvious precipitating cause. Secondary aplastic anaemia may result from a variety of industrial, accidental, iatrogenic and infectious causes (Table 5.1).

Table 5.1 Causes of aplastic anaemia.

PRIMARY   Congenital (Fanconi and non-Fanconi types)
          Idiopathic acquired

SECONDARY (I) *Ionising radiations:* radiology, radiotherapy, radioactive isotopes, nuclear power stations
          (II) *Chemicals:* benzene and other organic solvents, TNT, insecticides, hair dyes, chlordane, DDT
          Drugs: which regularly cause marrow depression (e.g. busulphan, cyclophosphamide, chlorambucil, vinblastine, 6-mercaptopurine, etc.); *which occasionally or rarely cause marrow depression* (e.g. chloramphenicol, sulphonamides, phenylbutazone, gold, and others)
          (III) *Infection:* viral hepatitis (A or non-A, non-B)

Pathogenesis

The underlying defect in all cases appears to be a substantial reduction in the numbers of haemopoietic pluripotential stem cells, and a fault in the remaining stem cells which makes them unable to divide and differentiate sufficiently to repopulate the marrow. A primary fault in the marrow microenvironment has also been suggested but the success of bone marrow transplantation shows this can only be a rare cause since normal donor stem cells are usually able to thrive in the recipient's marrow cavity. In some cases a cell-mediated immune mechanism is present (see below).

CONGENITAL

The Fanconi type has a recessive inheritance pattern (e.g. resulting from the marriage of first-cousins) and is often associated with other congenital defects of, for example, the skeleton, renal tract or skin; sometimes there is mental retardation. There are chromosomal abnormalities (random breaks). Some congenital cases (non-Fanconi) do not show these other defects or chromosome changes.

Sm. Thumb.
Sm Head .
Hypoplastic Radius
Syndactylly.

leukaemia

IDIOPATHIC ACQUIRED

In some cases, an auto-immune mechanism in which the patient's T-lymphocytes are thought to suppress haemopoietic stem cells seems likely, on the basis of in-vitro marrow culture experiments and clinical response to intense immunosuppression with, for example, anti-thymocyte globulin, high doses of corticosteroids or cyclophosphamide. In other cases (approximately 50%), there is no definite evidence for this or any other immune, infectious or metabolic cause. A defect of the marrow stem cells which limits their proliferative capacity seems likely.

SECONDARY

This is often due to direct damage to the haemopoietic marrow by radiation or cytotoxic drugs. The antimetabolite drugs (e.g. methotrexate) and mitotic inhibitors (e.g. daunorubicin) cause only temporary aplasia but the alkylating agents, particularly busulphan, may cause chronic aplasia closely resembling the chronic idiopathic disease. In these cases, the drugs are known to be marrow depressants and often large doses have been given for prolonged periods. Some individuals develop aplastic anaemia, however, when exposed to drugs such as phenylbutazone (see Table 5.1) which are not known to be cytotoxic or they may develop the disease during or within a few months of illness with infectious hepatitis. Because the incidence of marrow toxicity is particularly high for chloramphenicol, this drug should be reserved for treatment of those infections which are life-threatening (e.g. typhoid) and for which it is the optimum antibiotic. Chronic benzene exposure usually causes a hypercellular dyserythropoietic marrow (in which the erythroblasts show many bizarre features such as binuclearity, nuclear bridging, megaloblastosis) but may occasionally cause a true aplastic anaemia.

CLL.

Clinical features

The onset is at any age with a peak incidence around 30 and a slight male predominance; it can be insidious or acute with symptoms and signs resulting from anaemia, neutropenia or thrombocytopenia. Infections, particularly of the mouth and throat, are common and generalised infections are frequently life-threatening; ecchymoses, bleeding gums, epistaxes and menorrhagia are the most frequent haemorrhagic manifestations and the usual presenting features often with symptoms of anaemia. The lymph nodes, liver and spleen are not enlarged.

Laboratory findings

(i)   Anaemia is normochromic, normocytic or macrocytic (MCV often 95–110 fl). The reticulocyte count is reduced and extremely low in relation to the degree of anaemia.

(ii)   Leucopenia. There is a selective fall in granulocytes, usually but not always below $1.5 \times 10^9/l$. In severe cases, the lymphocyte count is also low. The neutrophils appear normal and their alkaline phosphatase score is high.

(iii)   Thrombocytopenia is always present and, in severe cases, is less than $10 \times 10^9/l$.

(iv)   There are no abnormal cells in the peripheral blood.

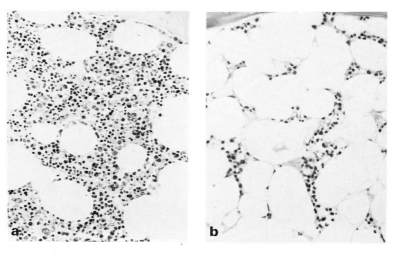

Fig. 5.1a   Normal iliac crest bone marrow trephine.

Fig. 5.1b   Aplastic (hypoplastic) anaemia iliac crest bone marrow trephine.

(v)   Bone marrow shows hypoplasia, with loss of haemopoietic tissue and replacement by fat which comprises over 75% of the marrow. Trephine biopsy is essential and may show patchy cellular areas in a hypocellular background (Fig. 5.1). The main cells present are lymphocytes and plasma cells; megakaryocytes in particular are reduced or absent.

Aplastic anaemia and anaemia in systemic diseases   89

Diagnosis

The disease must be distinguished from other causes of pancyto-penia (Table 5.2) and this is not usually difficult provided an adequate bone marrow sample is obtained. In some centres, ferro-kinetic studies with labelled iron (^{59}Fe) are performed. These show

Table 5.2 Causes of pancytopenia.

1 Aplastic anaemia (including cytotoxic drug therapy)
2 Bone marrow infiltration (e.g. carcinoma, tuberculosis, lymphoma)
3 Leukaemia, some myelodysplastic syndromes, myeloma
4 Hypersplenism (e.g. portal hypertension, lipidoses, e.g. Gaucher's disease, Felty's syndrome)
5 Megaloblastic anaemia
6 Myelosclerosis (some cases)
7 Paroxysmal nocturnal haemoglobinuria (some cases)

slow clearance of the isotope from the blood stream, poor uptake by the marrow, and subsequent inadequate incorporation into circulating red cells (Fig. 5.2). Most of the iron accumulates in the liver. If the reticulocyte count is raised, paroxysmal noctural haemoglobinuria must be excluded by examination of urine for haemosiderin and by the acid lysis tests.

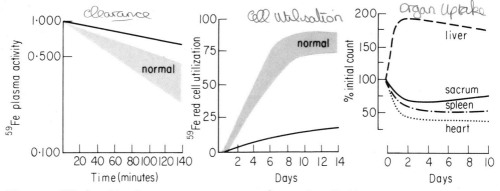

Fig. 5.2 ^{39}Fe ferrokinetic study in aplastic anaemia showing: (*Left*) Slow clearance of ^{59}Fe; (*centre*) grossly reduced ^{59}Fe red cell utilisation; and (*right*) surface counting evidence of liver uptake of ^{59}Fe and impaired bone marrow (sacral) uptake. Shaded areas = normal range.

Treatment and prognosis

The cause, if known, is removed, e.g. radiation or drug therapy discontinued. Initial management largely consists of support care with blood transfusions, platelet concentrates and treatment and prevention of infection. In very severely thrombocytopenic (plate-let count $< 10 \times 10^9$/l) or neutropenic (neutrophils $< 0.5 \times 10^9$/l) patients, management is similar to the support care of acute leukaemia (p. 133). An antifibrinolytic agent (e.g. tranexamic acid) may be used in patients with severe prolonged thrombocytopenia. Recently, the use of an oral antifungal agent (e.g. amphotericin, ketoconazole or mycostatin) together with co-trimoxazole has been advocated to prevent systemic infection by fungi.

The choice of more specific therapy depends partly on correct assessment of the patient's chance of spontaneous recovery. In the most severe cases, assessed by reticulocyte, neutrophil and platelet counts and degree of loss of marrow haemopoietic tissue, the chance of survival beyond 6–12 months is less than 50%. Cases following viral hepatitis fall into this group. Less severe cases may have an acute transient course, or a chronic course with ultimate recovery, although the platelet count often remains subnormal for many years. Relapses, sometimes severe and occasionally fatal, may also occur and, rarely, the disease transforms into acute leukaemia or paroxysmal nocturnal haemoglobinuria (p. 85).

Table 5.3 Bone marrow transplantation (allogeneic).

Indications
Some cases of:
	Severe aplastic anaemia
	Acute leukaemia (current trials)
	   AML in first remission
	   ALL in second remission
	Chronic granulocytic leukaemia in chronic phase
	Rare inherited disorders, e.g. combined immunodeficiency disease, Hurler's syndrome, glycogen storage disease, osteopetrosis, thalassaemia major

Donor	HLA, mixed lymphocyte culture (MLC) matched sibling ('allogeneic') Identical twin ('syngeneic') Unrelated but HLA, MLC matched donor
Preparation of recipient	Massive doses of cyclophosphamide on days 5, 4, 3, 2 before transplant (modify and add total body irradiation in leukaemia)
Technique	Harvest at least 10^9 nucleated marrow cells (500–1000 ml) from donor by multiple aspiration, filter and infuse intravenously into recipient
Post-transplant management	General support measures e.g. platelets, prevent infections with gut and skin decontamination, laminar airflow isolation Intermittent methotrexate or cyclosporin A to prevent graft-versus-host disease unless donor T cells removed at transplant
Main complications	Graft-versus-host disease (GVHD) Graft rejection Severe infections, pneumonitis

The following 'specific' treatments have been attempted with varied success:

Androgens. Orally administered androgens (e.g. methanedione or oxymetholone) have been used in high doses for at least 3–6 months and, although controlled trials have not confirmed an overall improved prognosis, there is no doubt that some cases have improved. Side-effects include salt retention, cholestatic jaundice, a hepatitic picture or, rarely, hepatocellular carcinoma. Virilisation is also a problem in females and children.

High dose corticosteroids. Responses to methyl prednisolone, 2 g daily, have been reported but are unusual.

Anti-thymocyte (anti-lymphocyte) globulin. This has been used with benefit in about 50% of cases in controlled trials. The mechanism may be elimination of suppressor or killer T-cells thought to be damaging haemopoietic stem cells. Side-effects include febrile reactions, thrombocytopenia and serum sickness.

Bone marrow transplantation (Table 5.3). This involves repopulating the bone marrow of a recipient with the pluripotent stem cells of a donor. These donor stem cells ultimately provide the recipient with new haemopoietic and lymphoid systems. The recipient marrow and lymphoid system is destroyed prior to the transplantation either by massive chemotherapy (e.g. with cyclophosphamide (Fig. 5.3)) or, in the case of leukaemia, with total body irradiation and chemotherapy aimed also at destroying all residual leukaemic cells. The donor marrow cells are infused intravenously and seed the marrow cavity but not other organs. A period of severe pancytopenia of about 21 days—during which the patient must be protected from infections or haemorrhage—precedes the appearance of mature donor cells in the peripheral blood. The donor is usually an HLA-identical, MLC-unreactive sibling or an identical twin. Bone marrow transplantation is performed most commonly in the treatment of leukaemia (see p. 139) but may also be used to treat aplastic anaemia and a variety of hereditary conditions (see Table 5.3). It is considered in severe cases of aplastic anaemia under the age of 50, where an HLA and mixed lymphocyte culture matching sibling is available and the prognosis without transplantation is > 50% mortality. If the patient has an identical twin (syngeneic), bone marrow transplantation is undertaken even in less severe cases. The success rate of allogeneic transplantation in aplastic anaemia is now 60–70% long-term survivors. Cyclosporin A is used to reduce the severity of graft-versus-host disease and also to prevent acute graft rejection. A typical satisfactory response is shown in Fig. 5.3. Death during or after transplantation may be due to overwhelming infection, particularly if there is graft rejection, or to acute or chronic graft-versus-host disease. This is thought to be due to donor T-

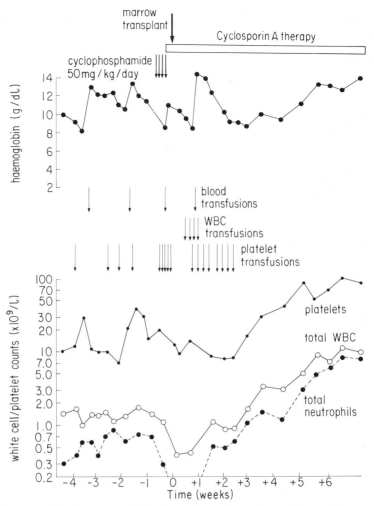

Fig. 5.3 The haematological chart of a patient who underwent bone marrow transplantation for aplastic anaemia. The donor was a sibling (allogeneic transplantation). Prior to bone marrow transplantation for acute leukaemia, it is usual to give cyclophosphamide for two days only followed by total body irradiation and in some centres, methotrexate is given rather than cyclosporin, or donor T cells are removed in vitro with antibodies at the time of transplantation.

Donor T – lymphocytes reacting against host tissues and is manifested by erythematous skin reactions, liver dysfunction and severe gastrointestinal disease with marked diarrhoea. The disease is assessed according to clinical and histological severity into four grades.

Pure red cell aplasia

This is a rare syndrome characterised by anaemia with normal leucocytes and platelets and grossly reduced or absent erythroblasts from the marrow. It may be congenital (Diamond–Blackfan syndrome) or acquired. Parvovirus infection causes a transient red cell aplasia which results in severe anaemia in patients with pre-existing shortened red cell survival, e.g. sickle cell disease or hereditary spherocytosis. The acquired form may also occur with no obvious associated disease or precipitating factor ('idiopathic'), or in association with autoimmune diseases (especially SLE), with a thymoma or lymphoma. In some cases immunosuppression is helpful, while in the congenital variety, corticosteroids or androgens may produce improvement in the anaemia but the long-term effects on growth are a serious side-effect of the prolonged use of these drugs in infancy and childhood.

ANAEMIA IN SYSTEMIC DISEASE

Many of the anaemias seen in clinical practice occur in patients with common systemic disorders and are the result of a number of contributing factors. Many of these factors are common to several diseases (e.g. the anaemia of chronic disorders, iron deficiency, folate deficiency), but some are particularly associated with one or other system. The factors causing anaemia in some of these various diseases of organs other than the bone marrow are summarised briefly below.

Malignant disease

Contributing factors include: anaemia of chronic disorders, (p. 38), blood loss, marrow infiltration (with a leuco-erythroblastic blood picture) (p. 108), folate deficiency, haemolysis (e.g. microangiopathic or auto-immune), marrow suppression from radiotherapy or chemotherapy, renal disease and hypersplenism.

Rheumatoid arthritis (and other connective tissue disorders)

Contributory factors include: anaemia of chronic disorders, blood loss (especially following chronic aspirin ingestion), marrow aplasia (due to analgesic drugs, e.g. phenylbutazone or gold), folate deficiency, hypersplenism (Felty's syndrome), and auto-immune haemolysis (particularly in SLE).

Chronic renal failure

The main contributing factors include: reduced erythropoietin production, the anaemia of chronic disorders, and haemolysis with 'burr' cells (Fig. 1.17a). There is approximately a 2 g/dl fall in haemoglobin for every 10 mmol/l rise in blood urea. Additional factors in some patients are: blood loss, microangiopathic haemolysis, and folate deficiency.

Liver disease and alcohol

Contributing factors include: blood loss (e.g. bleeding varices), hypersplenism, liver disease itself (this is associated with macrocytes and target cells), haemolysis (auto-immune haemolytic anaemia which occasionally occurs with chronic active hepatitis), *Aplastic A* folate deficiency, and alcohol (which may have a direct toxic action on the marrow and result in macrocytosis; it is occasionally associated with sideroblastic change). Rarely an acute haemolytic anaemia associated with hyperlipidaemia follows a particularly heavy intake of alcohol (Zieve's syndrome).

Patients with liver disease are more likely to bleed because of thrombocytopenia due to hypersplenism, antibodies to platelets or to disseminated intravascular coagulation, or because of deficiency of clotting factors II, VII, IX and X (vitamin K-dependent) and, in advanced liver disease, factor V, which is also synthesised by the liver. Abnormalities of platelet and fibrinogen function may also be present.

Hypothyroidism

This anaemia may be due to lack of thyroxine. There is reduced O_2 need and thus reduced erythropoietin secretion. The anaemia is often macrocytic and the MCV falls with thyroxine therapy. Hypothyroidism may be associated with pernicious anaemia; iron deficiency may also be present.

Tuberculosis

The dominant factor in the pathogenesis of anaemia in tuberculosis is the anaemia of chronic disorders. Other factors include: marrow replacement by tuberculosis which may occur with miliary disease; anti-tuberculous drug therapy (e.g. isoniazid is a pyridoxine antagonist and may cause sideroblastic anaemia).

→ Haemolytic Anaemia with G6PDD deficiency

Drugs

Abnormalities of the blood are among the most frequent side effects of many drugs. These are discussed in the appropriate chapters and include marrow aplasia, selective neutropenia or thrombocytopenia, haemolytic anaemias of various types, megaloblastic anaemia, sideroblastic anaemia, and abnormalities of platelet and phagocyte function.

Erythrocyte sedimentation rate (ESR)

This commonly used but non-specific test measures the speed of rouleaux formation and sedimentation of red cells in plasma over a period of one hour. The speed is mainly dependent on the plasma concentration of large proteins, e.g. fibrinogen and immuno-globulins. The normal range in men is 1-5 mm per hour and in women 5-15 mm per hour and there is a progressive increase in old age. The ESR is raised in a wide variety of systemic inflammatory and neoplastic diseases and in pregnancy. The highest values (> 100 mm per hour) are found in chronic infections, including tuberculosis and Kala azar, myeloma and macroglobulinaemia, connective tissue disorders and disseminated cancer. A raised ESR is associated with marked rouleaux formation of red cells in the peripheral blood film (see Fig. 9.4). The ESR can be used to monitor the response to therapy. In some laboratories, measurement of ESR has been replaced by plasma viscosity determination.

SELECTED BIBLIOGRAPHY

Buckner C.D. et al (1981) Bone marrow transplantation. In Recent Advances in Haematology 3, ed. A.V. Hoffrand. Churchill Livingstone, Edinburgh.

Camitta B.M. et al (1982) Aplastic anemia. New England Journal of Medicine 306, 645-52. 712-18.

Clinics in Haematology (1978) vol. 7.3, Aplastic Anemia. Ed. E.D. Thomas. W.B. Saunders, Philadelphia.

Clinics in Haematology (1983) vol. 12.3, Bone Marrow Transplantation. Ed. D.G. Nathan. W.B. Saunders, Philadelphia.

de Gruchy G.C. (1975) Drug-Induced Blood Disorders. Blackwell Scientific Publications, Oxford.

Gale R.P. et al (1981) Aplastic anemia. Annals of Internal Medicine 95, 477-94.

Geary C.G. (Ed.) (1979) Aplastic Anaemia. Ballière Tindall, London.

Girdwood R.H. (1973) Blood Disorders due to Drugs and other Agents. Excerpta Medica, London.

Gordon-Smith E.C. (1983) Management of aplastic anaemia. British Journal of Haematology 53, 185-8.

Israels M.C.G. & Delamore I.W. (Eds.) (1976) Haematological Aspects of System Disease. W.B. Saunders, Philadelphia.

Lewis S.M. & Verwilghen R.L. (Eds.) (1977) Dyserythropoiesis. Academic Press, London.

Major textbooks of haematology (see Chapter 1).

Chapter 6
The white cells

The white blood cells (leucocytes) may be divided into two broad groups—the phagocytes and the lymphocytes.

Granulocytes, which include three types of cell, neutrophils (polymorphs), eosinophils and basophils, together with monocytes comprise the phagocytes. The lymphocytes, their precursor cells, and plasma cells make up the immunocyte population. Normally only mature phagocytic cells and lymphocytes are found in the peripheral blood (Table 6.1, Fig. 6.1).

Table 6.1 White cells: normal blood counts.

Adults	
Total leucocytes	$4.00–11.0 \times 10^9/l^\star$
Neutrophils	$2.50–7.5 \times 10^9/l^\star$
Eosinophils	$0.04–0.4 \times 10^9/l$
Monocytes	$0.20–0.8 \times 10^9/l$
Basophils	$0.01–0.1 \times 10^9/l$
Lymphocytes	$1.50–3.5 \times 10^9/l$
Children	
Total leucocytes	
Neonates	$10.0–25.0 \times 10^9/l$
1 year	$6.0–18.0 \times 10^9/l$
4–7 years	$6.0–15.0 \times 10^9/l$
8–12 years	$4.5–13.5 \times 10^9/l$

$\star$ Normal Black and Middle-Eastern subjects may have lower counts.

The function of phagocytes and immunocytes in protecting the body against infection is closely connected with two soluble protein systems of the body, immunoglobulins and complement. These proteins, which may also be involved in blood cell destruction in a number of diseases, are discussed in this chapter.

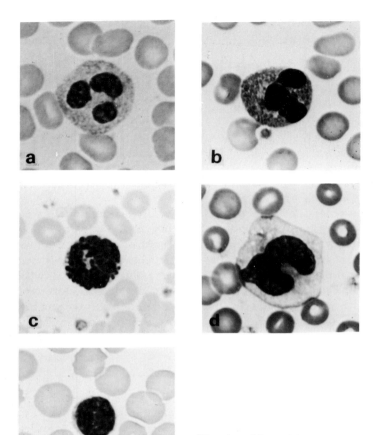

Fig. 6.1 Normal leucocyte
appearances **a** neutrophil
(polymorph), **b** eosinophil,
c basophil, **d** monocyte,
e lymphocyte.

Normal leucocyte appearance

NEUTROPHIL (POLYMORPH)

This cell 12–15 μm in diameter has a characteristic dense nucleus
consisting of between 2 and 5 lobes and a pale cytoplasm with
an irregular outline and containing many fine pink (azurophilic)
or violet-pink granules (see Fig. 6.1a). The granules are divided
into primary which appear in the promyelocyte stage, and secondary which appear at the myelocyte stage and predominate in the
mature neutrophil. Both granules are lysosomal in origin, the primary contains myeloperoxidase, acid phosphatase and other acid
hydrolases, the secondary contains alkaline phosphatase and
lysosyme.

These do not normally appear in peripheral blood but are present in the marrow (Fig. 6.2). The earliest recognisable precursor is the myeloblast, a cell of variable size (10–20 μm in diameter) which has a large nucleus with fine chromatin and usually 2–5 nucleoli. The cytoplasm is basophilic and no cytoplasmic granules are present. The normal bone marrow contains up to 4% of myeloblasts. Myeloblasts give rise by cell division to promyelocytes which are slightly larger cells which have developed primary granules in the cytoplasm. These cells give rise to myelocytes which have specific or secondary granules. The nuclear chromatin is now more condensed and nucleoli are not visible. Separate myelocytes of the eosinophil and basophil series can be identified. The myelocytes give rise by cell division to metamyelocytes, non-dividing cells, which have an indented or horseshoe-shaped nucleus and cytoplasm filled with primary and secondary granules. Most workers classify a stage of neutrophil maturation between the metamyelocytes and fully mature neutrophils as 'band' or 'juvenile' forms. These cells which may occur in normal peripheral blood do not contain the clear fine filamentous distinction between lobes which is seen in the mature neutrophils.

MONOCYTES

These are of variable appearance, usually larger than other peripheral blood leucocytes (16–20 μm in diameter) and possess a large central oval or indented nucleus with clumped chromatin (see Fig. 6.1d). The abundant cytoplasm stains pale blue and contains many fine vacuoles giving a ground-glass appearance. Cytoplasmic granules are also often present. The monocyte precursors in the marrow (monoblasts and promonocytes) are difficult to distinguish from myeloblasts and monocytes.

EOSINOPHILS

These cells are similar to neutrophils except the cytoplasmic granules are coarser and more deeply red staining (since they contain a basic protein) and there are rarely more than three nuclear lobes (see Fig. 6.1b). Eosinophil myelocytes can be recognised but earlier stages are indistinguishable from neutrophil precursors. The blood transit time for eosinophils is longer than for neutrophils. They enter inflammatory exudates and appear to have a special role in allergic responses, in defence against parasites and in removal of fibrin formed during inflammation.

BASOPHILS

These are only occasionally seen in normal peripheral blood. They have many cytoplasmic granules which overlie the nucleus and contain heparin and histamine (see Fig. 6.1c). In the tissues they become mast cells. They have IgE attachment sites and their degranulation is associated with histamine release.

LYMPHOCYTES

Most lymphocytes present in the peripheral blood are small cells less than 10 μm in diameter. Their deeply staining nuclei are round or slightly indented with coarse, ill-defined aggregates of chromatin (see Fig 6.1e). Nucleoli are not normally seen. The cytoplasm stains sky-blue and, in most cells, is seen as a scanty rim around the nucleus. About 10% of circulating lymphocytes are larger cells 12–16 μm in diameter with more abundant cytoplasm which may contain a few azurophilic granules. These larger forms are believed to have been stimulated by antigenic challenge, e.g. viruses or foreign proteins. Lymphocyte production and development is discussed later in this chapter.

Granulocyte formation and kinetics

The blood granulocytes and monocytes are formed in the bone marrow from a common precursor cell (Fig. 6.2). In the granulopoietic series the myeloblast, the promyelocyte and the myelocyte form a proliferative or mitotic pool of cells while the metamyelocytes, band and segmented granulocytes make up a post-mitotic maturation compartment (Fig. 6.2). Large numbers of band and segmented neutrophils are also held in the marrow as a 'reserve pool' or storage compartment. The bone marrow normally contains more myeloid cells than erythroid cells in the ratio of 2 : 1–12 : 1, the largest proportion being neutrophils and metamyelocytes. In the stable or normal state, the bone marrow storage compartment contains 10–15 times the number of granulocytes found in the peripheral blood. Following their release from the bone marrow, granulocytes spend about 10 hours in the circulation before moving into the tissues where they perform their phagocytic function. In the blood stream there are two pools of about equal size — the circulating pool (included in the blood count) and the marginating pool (not included in the blood count). It has been estimated that they spend on average 4–5 days in the tissues before they are destroyed during defensive action or as the result of senescence.

To control the various compartments of granulocyte renewal it is assumed that there is a feedback system between circulating and tissue granulocytes and the marrow (Fig. 6.3). These are

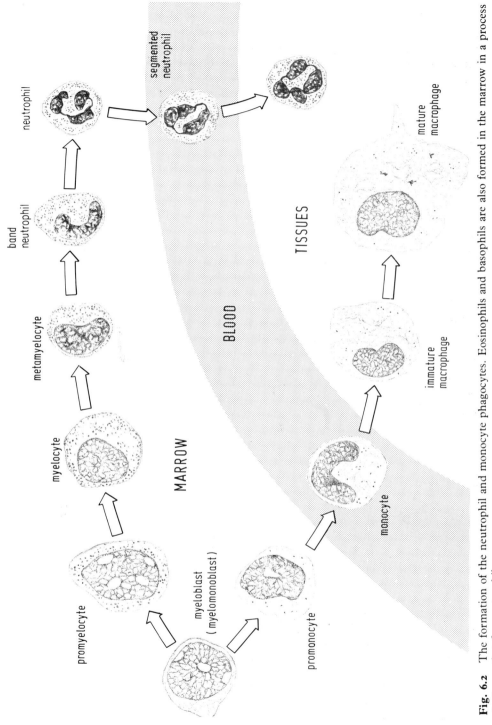

Fig. 6.2 The formation of the neutrophil and monocyte phagocytes. Eosinophils and basophils are also formed in the marrow in a process similar to that for neutrophils.

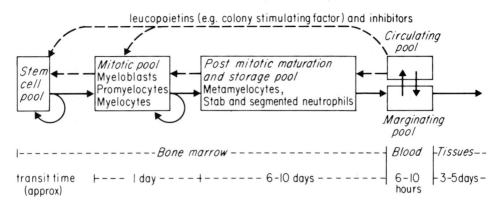

Fig. 6.3 Neutrophil granulocyte kinetics. Modified from Boggs & Winkelstein (1978).

stimulating factors ('leucopoietins') analogous to erythropoietin. Studies of in-vitro granulocyte colony formation in semi-solid agar culture have identified the presence of 'colony stimulating activities' (CSAs) in plasma, urine and locally in the marrow which may represent leucopoietins or their breakdown products. Feedback inhibitors of granulopoiesis also exist.

Monocyte formation and kinetics

Monocytes spend only a short time in the marrow and, after circulating for 20–40 hours, leave the blood to enter the tissues where they mature and carry out their principal functions. Their extravascular lifespan after their transformation to macrophages may be as long as several months or even years. They may assume specific functions in different tissues, e.g. skin, gut, liver, etc.

Neutrophil and monocyte function

The normal function of neutrophils and monocytes may be divided into three phases:

1 *Chemotaxis* (cell mobilisation and migration) in which the phagocyte is attracted to bacteria or site of inflammation probably by chemotactic substances released from damaged tissues or by complement components.

2 *Phagocytosis* in which the foreign material (e.g. bacteria, fungi, etc.) or dead or damaged cells of the host's body are phagocytosed. Recognition of a foreign particle is aided by opsonisation with immunoglobulin or complement since both neutrophils and monocytes have surface receptors for the Fc fragment of immunoglobulins and for C_3 and other complement components. Opsonisation of normal body cells (e.g. red cells or platelets) also makes them liable to destruction by macrophages of the RE system, as

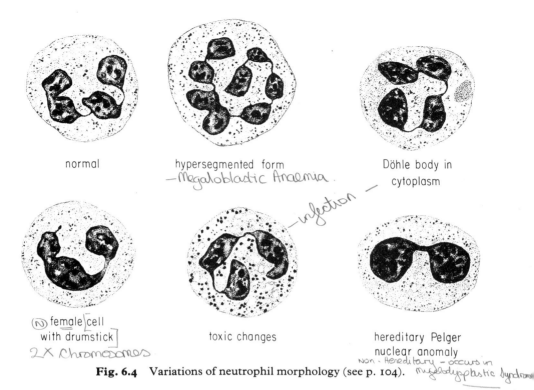

normal

hypersegmented form
—Megaloblastic Anaemia.

Döhle body in
cytoplasm

— infection —

(N) female cell
with drumstick
2X Chromosomes

toxic changes

hereditary Pelger
nuclear anomaly
Non · Hereditary – occurs in

Fig. 6.4 Variations of neutrophil morphology (see p. 104). myelodysplastic syndrome

in auto-immune haemolysis, idiopathic (auto-immune) thrombocytopenic purpura or many of the drug-induced cytopenias.
Macrophages also have a role in presenting foreign antigens to the
immune system.

3 *Killing and digestion.* This occurs by oxygen-dependent and
oxygen-independent pathways. In the oxygen-dependent reactions, super-oxide and hydrogen peroxide (H_2O_2), are generated
from oxygen and NADPH or NADH. In neutrophils, H_2O_2 reacts
with myeloperoxidase and intracellular halide to kill bacteria;
superoxide (O_2^-) may also be involved. The non-oxidative microbi-
cidal mechanism involves a fall in pH within phagocytic vacuoles
into which lysosomal enzymes are released. An additional factor,
lactoferrin—an iron binding protein present in neutrophil granules—is bacteriostatic by depriving bacteria of iron.

Defects of phagocytic cell function

1 *Chemotactic.* These occur in rare congenital abnormalities
(e.g. 'lazy leucocyte' syndrome, complement abnormalities) and
in more common acquired abnormalities either of the environment,
e.g. corticosteroid therapy, hypophosphataemia, aspirin, alcohol,
high plasma osmolarity (as in diabetes), or of the leucocytes themselves, e.g. in myeloid leukaemias and myelodysplastic syndromes.

The white cells 103

2   *Phagocytic.* These usually arise because of lack of opsonisation which may be due to congenital or acquired causes of hypogammaglobulinaemia, to lack of complement components or to lack of a serum factor which stimulates phagocytosis ('tuftsin') as after splenectomy or in sickle cell disease.

3   *Killing.* This is clearly illustrated by the rare X-linked recessive chronic granulomatous disease which results from abnormal leucocyte oxidative metabolism, probably due to one of several different enzyme defects.

Other rare congenital abnormalities may also result in defects of bacterial killing, e.g. myeloperoxidase deficiency and the Chediak–Higashi syndrome. Acute myeloblastic leukaemia, chronic granulocytic leukaemia and myelodysplastic syndromes may also be associated with defective killing of ingested microorganisms.

Variations in neutrophil morphology

Fig. 6.4 shows some of the more common abnormalities of neutrophil morphology which can be seen in the peripheral blood. Hypersegmented forms occur in megaloblastic anaemia, Döhle bodies and toxic changes in infection. The 'drumstick' appears on the nucleus of a proportion of the neutrophils in normal females and is due to the presence of two X chromosomes.

Neutrophil leucocytosis

An increase in circulating neutrophils to levels greater than $7.5 \times 10^9/l$ is one of the most frequently observed blood count changes (Table 6.2). Neutrophil leucocytosis is often accompanied by fever due to the release of leucocyte pyrogen. Other characteristic features of reactive neutrophilia (Table 6.2, 1–5) include **a**   a 'shift to the left' in the peripheral blood differential white cell count, i.e. an increase in the number of band forms and the occasional presence of more primitive cells such as metamyelocytes and myelocytes; **b**   the presence of cytoplasmic toxic granulation and Döhle bodies (condensation of RNA) (Fig. 6.4); and **c**   an elevated neutrophil alkaline phosphatase score.   (↓ in CML)

Table 6.2   Causes of neutrophil leucocytosis.

1   Bacterial infections (especially pyogenic bacterial, localized or generalized)
2   Inflammation and tissue necrosis (e.g. myositis, vasculitis, cardiac infarct, trauma)
3   Metabolic disorders (e.g. uraemia, eclampsia, acidosis, gout)
4   Neoplasms of all types (e.g. carcinoma, lymphoma, melanoma)
5   Acute haemorrhage or haemolysis
6   Corticosteroid therapy
7   Myeloproliferative disease (e.g. chronic granulocytic leukaemia, polycythaemia vera, myelosclerosis)

Neutropenia

The lower limit of the normal neutrophil count is $2.5 \times 10^9/l$. When the absolute neutrophil level falls below $1.0 \times 10^9/l$ the patient is likely to have <u>recurrent infections</u> and when the count falls to less than $0.2 \times 10^9/l$ the risks are very serious. Neutropenia may be <u>selective or occur as part of a general pancytopenia</u> (Table 6.3). The possible mechanisms are illustrated in Fig. 6.5.

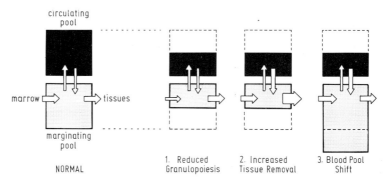

Fig. 6.5 Different kinetic mechanisms of neutropenia. Modified from Boggs & Winkelstein (1978).

DRUG-INDUCED NEUTROPENIA

Selective neutropenia may follow therapy with a large number of drugs (Table 6.3). Although in the majority the drug damages the

Table 6.3 Causes of neutropenia.

SELECTIVE NEUTROPENIA
—*Drug-induced:*
    Anti-inflammatory drugs (aminopyrine, phenylbutazone)
    Antibacterial drugs (chloramphenicol, co-trimoxazole)
    Anticonvulsants (phenytoin)
    Antithyroids (carbimazole)
    Hypoglycaemics (tolbutamide) (e Sulphonylurea)
    Phenothiazines (chlorpromazine, promethazine)
    Miscellaneous (mepacrine, phenindione and many others)
—*Benign* (racial or familial)
—*Cyclical*
—*Miscellaneous*
    Viral infections, e.g. hepatitis, influenza
    Fulminant bacterial infection, e.g. typhoid, miliary tuberculosis
    Hypersensitivity and anaphylaxis
    Auto-immune neutropenia
    Felty's syndrome
    Systemic lupus erythematosis

PART OF GENERAL PANCYTOPENIA
Bone marrow failure (see p. 90)
Splenomegaly

marrow precursor cell, a drug-hapten hypersensitivity affecting circulating neutrophils may be responsible in some cases, e.g. aminopyrine. An antibody is formed to a drug–protein complex acting as an antigen. Complement is bound and the immune complex and complement-coated neutrophils are rapidly removed from the circulation by RE cells.

CYCLICAL NEUTROPENIA

This is a rare syndrome with 3–4 week periodicity. Severe but temporary neutropenia occurs.

IDIOPATHIC BENIGN NEUTROPENIA

An increase in the marginating fraction of blood neutrophils and a corresponding reduction in the circulating fraction occurs in many normal Africans and other races and also, rarely, as a familial abnormality in other parts of the world. These subjects have no increased susceptibility to infection and their bone marrow appears normal.

[margin handwritten note: Racial or Familial]

CLINICAL FEATURES. Severe neutropenia is particularly associated with infections of the mouth and throat. Painful and often intractable ulceration may occur in these sites (Fig. 6.6), in the skin or at the anus. For other features of infections associated with severe neutropenia see p. 133.

DIAGNOSIS. Bone marrow examination is essential to determine whether there is depressed granulopoiesis with reduction in immature precursors or accelerated removal of circulating neutrophils when depletion of the bone marrow reserve of granulocytes leaves immature cells. This situation has erroneously been referred to as 'maturation arrest'. Marrow aspiration may also provide evidence of leukaemia or other infiltration.

MANAGEMENT. The treatment of patients with *acute severe neutropenia* is described on p. 133. In many patients with drug-induced neutropenia spontaneous recovery occurs within one or two weeks after stopping the drug.

Patients with *chronic neutropenia* have recurrent infections which are mainly bacterial in origin although fungal and viral infections (especially herpes) also occur. Early recognition and vigorous treatment with antibiotics, antifungal or antiviral agents as appropriate is essential. The role of prophylactic antibacterial agents, e.g. co-trimoxazole, is still undecided.

Corticosteroid therapy or splenectomy has been associated with good results in some patients with suspected *auto-immune neutropenia*, e.g. Felty's syndrome. On the other hand, cortico-

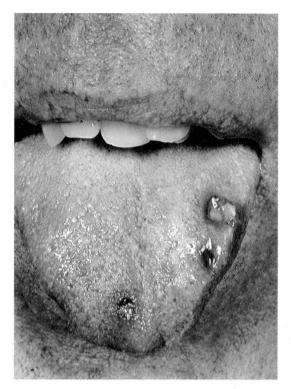

Fig. 6.6 Ulceration of the tongue in a patient with severe neutropenia.

steroids impair neutrophil function and should not be used indiscriminately in patients with neutropenia.

Eosinophilia

An increase in blood eosinophils above $0.4 \times 10^9/l$ occurs in:

1. Allergic diseases, especially hypersensitivity of the atopic type, e.g. bronchial asthma, hay fever, urticaria and food sensitivity.
2. Parasitic diseases, e.g. amoebiasis, hookworm, ascariasis, tapeworm infestation, filariasis, schistosomiasis and trichinosis.
3. Recovery from acute infection.
4. Certain skin diseases, e.g. psoriasis, pemphigus and dermatitis herpetiformis.
5. Pulmonary eosinophilia and the hyper-eosinophilic syndrome.
6. Drug sensitivity.
7. Polyarteritis nodosa.
8. Hodgkin's disease and some other tumours.
9. Eosinophilic leukaemia (rare).

Basophil leucocytosis

An increase in blood basophils above $0.1 \times 10^9/l$ is uncommon. The usual cause is a myeloproliferative disorder such as chronic granulocytic leukaemia or polycythemia vera. Reactive basophil increases are sometimes seen in myxoedema, during smallpox or chickenpox infection, and in ulcerative colitis.

Monocytosis

A rise in blood monocyte count above $0.8 \times 10^9/l$ is also infrequent. The following conditions may be responsible:

1 Chronic bacterial infections: tuberculosis, brucellosis, bacterial endocarditis, typhoid.
2 Protozoan diseases.
3 Chronic neutropenia.
4 Hodgkin's disease.
5 Myelomonocytic and monocytic leukaemia.

The leukaemoid reaction

The leukaemoid reaction is a reactive but excessive leucocytosis characterised by the presence of immature cells (e.g. blasts, promyelocytes and myelocytes) in the peripheral blood. The majority of leukaemoid reactions involve granulocytes but occasionally lymphocytic reactions occur.

Associated disorders include severe or chronic infections, severe haemolysis or metastatic cancer. Leukaemoid reactions are often particularly marked in children.

Granulocyte changes such as toxic granulation and Döhle bodies and a high neutrophil alkaline phosphatase score help to differentiate the leukaemoid reaction from chronic granulocytic leukaemia. The presence of a large proportion of myelocytes and of the Philadelphia chromosome help to confirm chronic granulocytic leukaemia.

Leuco-erythroblastic reaction

In the leuco-erythroblastic reaction, erythroblasts as well as primitive white cells are found in the peripheral blood (Fig. 6.7). This blood film appearance (which is due to extramedullary haemopoiesis or infiltration of the marrow) may occur in:

1 Myelosclerosis (myeloid metaplasia).
2 Myeloid leukaemias.
3 Marrow infiltration: carcinoma, fibrosis, tuberculosis, myeloma, lymphoma.
4 Severe haemorrhage, haemolysis, or megaloblastic anaemia.

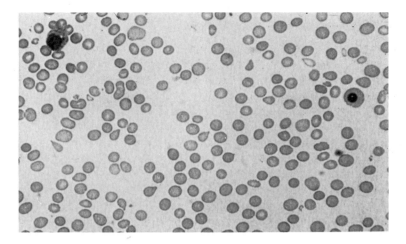

Fig. 6.7. The leuco-erythroblastic blood film reaction. The nucleated cells seen include an erythroblast and a myelocyte. The red cells show polychromasia, anisocytosis and poikilocytosis (including 'tear-drop' forms).

5 Lipidoses.
6 Marble bone disease (Albers-Schönberg, osteopetrosis).

LYMPHOCYTES

The immunologically competent cells or immunocytes comprise the lymphocytes, their precursors and plasma cells. These cells assist the phagocytes in the defence of the body against infection and other foreign invasion and they add specificity to the attack. Although a complete description of the functions of these cells is beyond the scope of this book, information essential to an understanding of the diseases of the lymphoid system, and of the role of lymphocytes in haematological diseases is included here.

Primary lymphocyte formation

In post-natal life the bone marrow and thymus are the primary lymphopoietic organs in which lymphocytic stem cells undergo spontaneous division not dependent upon antigenic stimulation (see Fig. 7.1). In the foetus, the yolk sac, liver and spleen are also lymphopoietic. The secondary or reactive lymphoid tissue is that found in the lymph nodes, the spleen, the organised and diffuse lymphoid tissues of the alimentary and respiratory tracts, together with the circulating lymphocytes in the blood and tissue spaces.

Functional aspects of lymphocytes—T- and B-cells

The immune response depends upon two types of lymphocytes, B- and T-cells (Table 6.4). In man, B-cells are derived from the bone marrow stem cells. Whether any of the cells are processed outside the bone marrow to become mature B-lymphocytes is uncertain. In birds this process takes place in the bursa of Fabricius but an equivalent organ has not been identified in man. After activation by antigens, B-cells proliferate and mature into plasma cells which secrete specific immunoglobulin antibodies. B-cells may also be instructed about specific antigens by circulating 'helper' T-cells, while macrophages play a role in processing many antigens before signalling in some way to B-lymphocytes to respond.

One of the most striking features of the immune system is its capacity to produce a highly specific response. For both T- and B-cells this specificity is achieved by the presence of receptors on the lymphocyte surface. The immune system contains many clones of lymphocytes. Each of these clones has a receptor which shows minor differences in structure from that of any other clone, and consequently will bind to different stimulating antigens. The variability is produced during B- or T-cell development by rearrangement of the immunoglobulin or T-cell receptor genes (see pp. 118-9). When an antigen is encountered only those clones to which the antigen binds are induced to proliferate and mature into effector cells—the phenomenon of clonal selection.

The B-cell receptor is essentially identical to the immunoglobulin it will secrete. The T-cell receptor is more complex. The portion that recognises antigen is structurally analogous to immunoglobulin, and has alpha and beta chains. T-cells, however, are unable to bind antigen free in solution and require it to be made available on specialised antigen presenting cells (APCs) found particularly in lymphoid tissues. Antigen on APCs is presented in association with molecules of the major histocompatibility complex (MHC) in man called HLA (see Fig. 14.3, p. 256). T-cells therefore must recognise not only the antigen, but also the 'self' MHC molecules. This capacity for MHC recognition appears to be the function of another component of the T-cell receptor, termed either the CD4 molecule in helper cells, which recognise Class 2 (HLA-DP, DQ and DR) molecules, or the CD8 molecule in cytotoxic effector cells, which recognise Class 1 (HLA A, B and C) molecules. The antigen recognition site and CD4 or CD8 molecule of the T-cell receptor appear to be joined together by a third component, CD3 (Fig. 6.8a).

Although the primary interaction between T-cells, B-cells and APCs is dependent on the presence of the appropriate antigen, the cells so activated then release amplification factors, called interleukin I and II and B-cell growth and differentiation factors

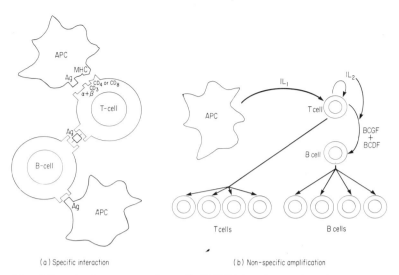

(a) Specific interaction   (b) Non-specific amplification

Fig. 6.8a Antigen presenting cells (APCs) bearing antigen interact with a T-cell with the appropriate receptor for the antigen and matching MHC molecules. B-cells with the appropriate surface receptor for the antigen are also stimulated. MHC recognition is, however, only needed for the primary activation of B-cells.

b Proliferation and differentiation of clones of the stimulated T- and B-cells result, under the influence of growth stimuli (interleukins [IL] I and II and B-cell growth and differentiation factors [BCGF and BCDF]).

which induce proliferation and differentiation in any activated clone (Fig. 6.8b).

It is not certain whether the thymus in humans is populated by cells (prothymocytes) derived directly from pluripotential bone marrow stem cells or from a bone marrow common lymphoid stem cell (Fig. 1.2). The primordial T-cells are conditioned by HLA-rich dendritic reticulum cells in the thymus and other tissues to recognise the body's own antigenic make up and to become the cells responsible for cell-mediated immunity. As well as helper (T_4) cells, the T-lymphocyte population includes suppressor (T_8) cells which reduce B-lymphocyte responses and cytotoxic cells which are capable of directly damaging cells recognised as foreign (*see* Fig. 7.1).

Further lymphocyte development—the germinal follicle

The B- and T-lymphocytes which leave the bone marrow and thymus respectively are 'virgin' cells, at an early stage of immunological maturation. When these T- and B-cells are presented with antigen by antigen-presenting cells for the first time, they transform into T- or B-immunoblasts (Fig. 6.8). The T-immunoblasts either carry out their primary T-cell function and die or they become 'memory' T-lymphocytes. These latter cells react more intensely and quickly during subsequent stimulation by the same antigen. B-immunoblasts give rise to plasma cells. Initially, these are small cells with features intermediate between those of typical small lymphocytes and typical mature plasma cells (plasmacytoid lymphocytes or lymphoplasmacytoid cells) and they secrete chiefly IgM. With further development they enlarge and become typical plasma cells which are responsible for the production of IgG, IgA, IgD and IgE. During the primary immune response the plasmacytoid lymphocytes predominate and the associated immunoglobulin production is small. Recent evidence suggests that bone marrow plasma cells may represent a different lineage from those in peripheral tissues (Fig. 7.1).

In the lymph nodes and other collections of lymphoid tissue, follicular germinal centres arise as a continuing response to antigenic stimulation. The typical dividing cells, known as centroblasts, arise from small lymphocytes and their progeny are known as centrocytes. These two types of lymphocytes are also known as follicle centre cells (FCC). Some of the centrocytes develop into memory cells of the B-cell system. The sequence of development of cells in follicular centres has not been established completely.

Lymphoblasts, as seen in lymphoblastic leukaemia or lymphoblastic lymphoma, cannot be distinguished by conventional microscopy from other early blast cells in a normal marrow, and are not identified in a normal germinal follicle. The cell is usually small with a diameter of 10–12 μm. The nucleus is usually rounded but may be convoluted. The chromatin pattern is fine and evenly dispersed with 1–5 inconspicuous nucleoli. The small amount of cytoplasm is only moderately basophilic. The morphological characteristics of lymphocytes have been described on p. 99. *Plasma cells* are larger than lymphocytes. Typically, they have an eccentric round nucleus with a 'clock-face' chromatin pattern. With the exception of a perinuclear light-staining Golgi body, the cytoplasm is strongly basophilic. *Immunoblasts* are the largest lymphoid cells. They have a light nucleus with fine chromatin pattern with very large nucleoli which are often solitary and found in the middle of the nucleus or at an indentation of the nuclear membrane. They have a broad rim of strongly basophilic cytoplasm. *Centroblasts* vary in size but are usually smaller than immunoblasts. The nucleus is round with a finely dispersed chromatin pattern with medium-sized nucleoli, which are often found at the inner nuclear membrane. Typically there is a rim of strongly basophilic cytoplasm. *Centrocytes* are small or medium-sized cells with round or conspicuous, notched, indented or deformed nuclei and weakly basophilic cytoplasm. Apart from their shape, the nuclei of these cells are easily distinguished from those of small lymphocytes in the mantle zone of the follicle by their light colour. Nucleoli, if present, are small and usually central.

Although reactive lymphoid cells are confined mainly to lymphoid tissues, they may also be seen in the blood in infectious mononucleosis (p. 115) and other infections (particularly viral) and during other immunological responses. In some of the malignant lymphomas (Chapter 8) there is blood involvement by the abnormal cells ('lymphosarcoma' or 'follicular lymphoma' cells). The germinal follicles also contain a network of dendritic reticulum cells and a few T-lymphocytes, mainly of the helper type.

Lymphocyte circulation

Lymphocytes in the peripheral blood migrate through post-capillary venules into the substance of the lymph nodes or into the spleen. T-cells home to the perifollicular zones of the cortical areas

Table 6.4 T- and B-lymphocytes — distinguishing features.

T-cells	B-cells
Responsible for cell mediated immunity (e.g. against intracellular organisms including many bacteria, viruses, protozoa and fungi; also against transplanted organs).	Responsible for humoral immunity (e.g. against encapsulated pyogenic bacteria).
Principal circulating population (80% of normal blood lymphocytes).	Majority are fixed and immobile (only 20% of normal blood lymphocytes).
Found in perifollicular areas of the deep cortex of lymph nodes, in periarteriolar tissue of the spleen and in the thymus. Divided into helper (T_{4+}) and suppressor (T_{8+}) which occupy different microenvironments.	Found in germinal centres of lymph nodes, spleen, alimentary and respiratory tract lymphoid aggregations. Also present in the superficial (subcapsular) cortical areas and medullary cords of lymph nodes.
Many long lived 'memory' cells but also short-lived cells.	Majority have short lifespan, e.g. plasma cells 2–3 days but also includes long-lived cells.
T specific surface membrane antigens.	Have surface immunoglobulins (SIg).*
Rosette with sheep RBC*.	Membrane receptors for Fc portion of IgG, immune complexes, and C_3 (EAC rosettes).
Mitogenic reaction with phytohaemagglutinin (PHA), pokeweed, heterologous leucocytes*.	Mitogenic reaction with endotoxin.

* = methods usually employed to detect T- and B-cells.

of lymph nodes (paracortical areas) (Fig. 7.1) and to the peri-arteriolar sheaths surrounding the central arterioles of the spleen. B-cells selectively accumulate in germinal follicles of the lymph nodes and spleen and also at the subcapsular periphery of the cortex and in the medullary cords of the lymph nodes. Lymphocytes return to the peripheral blood via the efferent lymphatic stream and the thoracic duct. The majority of the recirculating cells (e.g. in the thoracic duct or peripheral blood) are T-cells with a median duration of a complete circulation of about 10 hours (Table 6.4). The T-cells form two main subsets: suppressor (T_{8+}) and helper (T_{4+}). In normal peripheral blood and germinal centres, helper cells predominate but in the marrow and gut the major T-cell sub-population is suppressor. The majority of B-cells are more sessile and spend long periods in the spleen and lymph nodes.

Lymphocytosis

Lymphocytosis often occurs in infants and young children in response to infections which produce a neutrophil reaction in adults. Conditions particularly associated with lymphocytosis are listed in Table 6.5.

Table 6.5 Causes of lymphocytosis.

Infections
Acute—infectious mononucleosis, rubella, pertussis, acute infectious
         lymphocytosis, infectious hepatitis, cytomegalic virus
Chronic—tuberculosis, toxoplasmosis, brucellosis

Thyrotoxicosis

Chronic lymphocytic leukaemia (and some lymphomas)

Lymphopenia

Lymphopenia is uncommon, but may occur in severe bone marrow failure, with corticosteroid and other immunosuppressive therapy, in Hodgkin's disease and with widespread irradiation.

INFECTIOUS MONONUCLEOSIS

Infectious mononucleosis (glandular fever) is a disease characterised by fever, sore throat, lymphadenopathy and atypical lymphocytes in the blood. These are thought to be T-cells reacting against B-lymphocytes infected with Epstein–Barr (EB) virus. The condition is associated with a rising titre of antibody against the EB virus. Individuals without antibody to this virus are prone to the infection. As many people have antibodies without having had the obvious features of the disease, it appears likely that sub-clinical infection is common. There is a low infectivity rate. Sporadic groups of cases occur, particularly in young people living together in boarding schools, colleges and military institutions. The disease is associated with high titre of heterophile antibody reacting with sheep red cells. A similar clinical syndrome without heterophile antibodies may occur in young adults with toxoplasmosis or cytomegaloviral infections.

Clinical features

The majority of patients are between the ages of 15 and 40. A prodromal period of a few days occurs with lethargy, malaise, headaches, stiff neck and a dry cough. In established disease the following features may be found:
(i) Bilateral cervical lympadenopathy is present in 75% of cases. Symmetrical generalised lymphadenopathy occurs in 50% of cases. The nodes are discrete and may be tender.
(ii) Over half of patients have sore throats with inflamed oral and pharyngeal surfaces. Follicular tonsillitis is frequently seen.
(iii) Fever may be mild or severe.
(iv) A morbilliform rash, severe headache and eye signs, e.g. photophobia, conjunctivitis and periorbital oedema are not uncommon.
(v) Palpable splenomegaly occurs in over half the patients and hepatomegaly in about 15%.
(vi) About 5% of patients are jaundiced.
(vii) Occasionally in the most severely affected patients there is widespread mucosal bleeding with epistaxis, tachycardia with ECG abnormalities, or evidence of nervous system disease, e.g. convulsions, coma, stupor, various pareses or palsies involving cranial nerves or lower motor neurones. Involvement of mesenteric nodes may produce a clinical picture similar to that of acute appendicitis.

Diagnosis

1   *Pleomorphic atypical lymphocytosis.* A moderate rise in white cell count, e.g. $10-20 \times 10^9/l$ with an absolute lymphocytosis is usual, and some patients have even higher counts. Large numbers of atypical lymphocytes are seen in the peripheral blood film (Fig. 6.9). These cells are variable in appearance but most have nuclear and cytoplasmic features similar to those seen during reactive lymphocyte transformation. The greatest number of atypical lymphocytes are usually found between the 7th and 10th day of the illness and these cells may persist in the blood for one or two months.
2   *Heterophile antibodies.* Heterophile antibodies against sheep red cells may be found in the serum at high titres (Paul–Bunnell test). Similar antibodies are occasionally found in normals and were often seen in the past in patients suffering from serum sick-

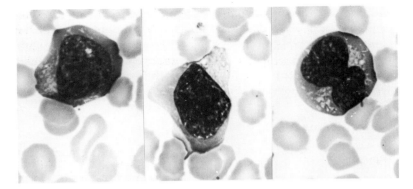

Fig. 6.9 Abnormal ('atypical') lymphocytes in the blood film in infectious mononucleosis. These are T-lymphocytes reacting against EB virus-infected B-lymphocytes.

ness. Differential absorption studies before the sheep cell titration allow distinction between these heterophile antibodies. Antibodies present in normals and those suffering from serum sickness are absorbed by a suspension of guinea-pig kidney which is rich in Forsmann antigen. The antibody in infectious mononucleosis is not absorbed by guinea-pig kidney but is absorbed by antigens on the membrane of ox red cells (Fig. 6.10). Highest titres occur during the second and third week and the antibody persists in most patients for six weeks. Modern slide screening tests in kit form substitute more sensitive formalised horse red cells for sheep cells.

3 *EB virus antibody.* If viral diagnostic facilities are available a rise in the titre of antibody against the EB virus may be demonstrated during the first two to three weeks.

Haematological abnormalities other than the atypical lympho-

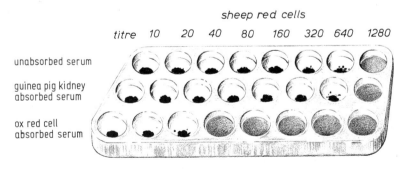

Heterophile antibody agglutination titres   unabsorbed serum = 640
GPK absorbed serum = 640
ox RBC absorbed serum = 40

ie ∶ Result consistent with infectious mononucleosis

Fig. 6.10 The Paul-Bunnell test for heterophile antibody.

cytosis are frequent. Occasional patients develop an auto-immune haemolytic anaemia. The IgM auto-antibody is typically of the 'cold' type and usually shows 'i' blood group specificity. An auto-immune thrombocytopenic purpura occurs in a smaller number of patients.

Patients with infectious mononucleosis may have false-positive serology for syphilis or rheumatoid arthritis.

DIFFERENTIAL DIAGNOSIS

The differential diagnosis includes a large number of conditions with similar clinical findings or blood film appearances. Apart from acute leukaemia, cytomegalovirus infection and toxoplasmosis, influenza, rubella, infectious hepatitis or follicular tonsillitis are most likely to create initial diagnostic confusion. In the rare condition of childhood known as acute infective lymphocytosis the fever is mild, there is no lymphadenopathy, splenomegaly or heterophile antibody.

Treatment

In the great majority of patients only symptomatic treatment is required. There is no evidence to suggest that either antibiotics or corticosteroids influence the course of the disease.

Course and prognosis

Most patients recover fully 4–6 weeks after initial symptoms. However, convalescence may be slow and associated with severe malaise and lethargy. Relapse occurs in about 6% of cases but almost all patients eventually recover. Isolated fatalities have resulted from encephalitis, oedema of the glottis, severe hepatic necrosis or splenic rupture.

IMMUNOGLOBULINS

These are a heterogenous group of proteins which are produced by plasma cells and B-lymphocytes and react with particular antigens. They are divided into five subclasses, IgG, IgA, IgM, IgD and IgE. IgG, the most common, contributes about 80% of normal serum immunoglobulin, and is further subdivided into four subclasses, IgG_1, IgG_2, IgG_3 and IgG_4. IgM is usually produced first in response to antigen, IgG subsequently and for a more prolonged period. IgA is the main immunoglobulin found in secretions, particularly of the gastrointestinal tract. IgD and IgE are minor fractions. Some important biochemical and biological properties of the three main immunoglobulin subclasses are summarised in Table 6.6.

Table 6.6 Some properties of the three main classes of immunoglobulin.

	IgG	IgA	IgM
Molecular weight	140 000	140 000	900 000
Sedimentation constant	7S	7S	19S
Normal serum level (g/l)	6.0–16.0	1.5–4.5	0.5–1.5
Present in	Serum and extracellular fluid	Serum and other body fluids, e.g. of bronchi and gut	Serum only
Complement fixation	Usual	No	Usual and very efficient
Placental transfer	Yes	No	No
Heavy chain	γ	α	μ

The immunoglobulins are all made up of the same basic structure (Fig. 6.11) consisting of two heavy chains (which are called gamma (γ), alpha (α), or mu (μ) in IgG, IgA and IgM respectively) and two light chains (kappa (κ) or lambda (λ)) which are common to all three immunoglobulins. IgM molecules are much larger because they consist of five subunits. The gene coding for components of immunoglobulins are situated on different chromosomes, heavy chain genes on chromosome 14, kappa chain genes on chromosome 2 and lambda genes on chromosome 22. During early B lymphocyte development immunoglobulin gene rearrangement takes place in developing B cells (Fig. 6.12).

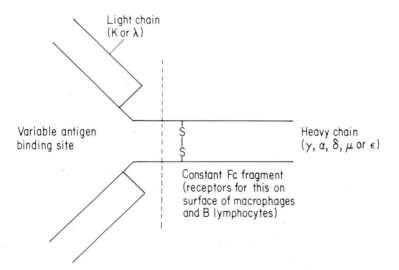

Light chain
(K or λ)

Variable antigen binding site

Heavy chain
(γ, α, δ, μ or ϵ)

Constant Fc fragment (receptors for this on surface of macrophages and B lymphocytes)

Fig. 6.11 The basic structure of the immunoglobulin molecule. IgA molecules tend to dimerize while IgM molecules consist of 5 subunits as in the diagram.

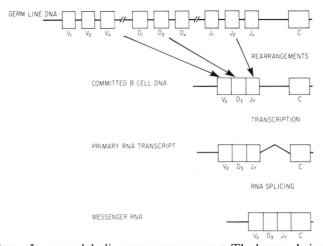

Fig. 6.12 Immunoglobulin gene rearrangement. The heavy-chains, kappa and lambda light-chain genes occur on chromosomes 14, 2 and 22 in man. In the embryonic germ-line state the heavy-chain genes occur as segments for variable (V), diversity (D), joining (J) and constant (C) regions. Each of the V, D and J segments contain a number (n) of different genes. In cells not committed to immunoglobulin synthesis, these gene segments remain in their germ-line state but during early differentiation of B-cells, there is rearrangement of heavy-chain genes so that one of the variable heavy-chain genes combines with one of the D genes and one of the J region genes which is adjacent to the constant region. They thus form an active transcriptional gene for the heavy chain. Diversity is introduced by the variability of which V segment joins with which D and which J segment. In this arbitrary example V_2 joins with D_3 and J_7. The constant region used may be gamma, alpha, mu, delta or epsilon. For the light-chains a similar rearrangement occurs with a variable light-chain segment joining with a J segment to form an active light-chain gene. Rearrangement occurs in the sequence heavy, kappa and lambda genes. In T-cells similar rearrangements to those of the immunoglobulin heavy-chain genes occur to generate diversity in the alpha and beta chains of the T-cell receptor.

The main role of immunoglobulins is defence of the body against foreign organisms. However, they also play a vital role in the pathogenesis of a number of haematological disorders. Secretion of a specific immunoglobulin from a monoclonal population of lymphocytes or plasma cells occurs in macroglobulinaemia and most cases of multiple myeloma. Bence-Jones protein found in the urine in some cases of myeloma consists of a monoclonal secretion of light chains (either kappa or lambda). Immunoglobulins may coat blood cells in a variety of immune or auto-immune haematological disorders and cause: **1** agglutination (e.g. in cold agglutinin disease, p. 82); **2** destruction by macrophages of the RE system (as in warm type auto-immune haemolytic anaemia or Rhesus disease of the newborn); or **3** complement coating of the cells which, in turn, may lead either to RE system destruction (as in many drug-induced immune disorders of blood cells) or to direct lysis if the complement sequence goes to completion (as in ABO incompatible blood transfusion).

COMPLEMENT

This consists of a series of serum globulins which are capable of lysis of bacteria or of blood cells or can 'opsonise' (coat) bacteria or cells so that they are phagocytosed. The complement sequence consists of nine major components — C_1, C_2, etc. — which are activated in turn (denoted thus $\overline{C_1}$) and form a cascade, resembling the coagulation sequence. The early (opsonising) stages leading

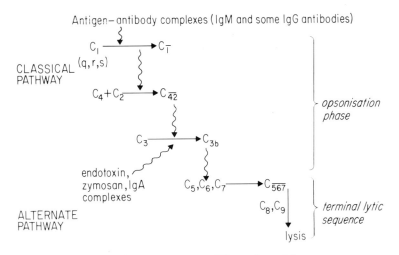

Fig. 6.13 The complement sequence. The activated factors are denoted by a bar over the number.

to coating the cells with C_{3b} can occur by two different pathways, the classical pathway usually activated by IgG or IgM coating of cells or the alternative, more rapid, pathway activated by IgA, endotoxin (from Gram-negative bacteria) and other factors (Fig. 6.13). Macrophages have C_3 receptors and they phagocytose C_3-coated cells. If the complement sequence goes to completion, there is generation of an active phospholipase that punches holes in the cell membrane (e.g. red cell or bacterial cell), causing direct lysis.

SELECTED BIBLIOGRAPHY

Boggs D.R. & Winkelstein A. (1978) *White Cell Manual*, 3rd edition. F.A. Davis, Philadelphia.
Cline M.J. (1975) *The White Cell*. Harvard University Press, Cambridge, Mass.

Cline M.J. & Golde D.W. (1977) Granulocytes and Monocytes: Function and Functional Disorders. In *Recent Advances in Haematology*, 2nd edition, eds. A.V. Hoffbrand, M.C. Brain and J. Hirsh. Churchill Livingstone, Edinburgh.

Clinics in Haematology (1979) vol. 8.2, Cellular Dynamics of Haemopoiesis. Ed. L. Lajtha. W.B. Saunders, Philadelphia.

Clinics in Haematology (1982) vol. 11.3, *The Lymphocytes*. Ed. G. Janossy. W.B. Saunders, Philadelphia.

Lachmann P.J. & Peters D.K. (1982) *Clinical Aspects of Immunology*, 5th edition. Blackwell Scientific Publications, Oxford.

Methods in Hematology (1981) *Leucocyte function*. Ed. M.J. Cline. Churchill Livingstone, Edinburgh.

Roitt I.M. (1984) *Essential Immunology*, 5th edition. Blackwell Scientific Publications, Oxford.

Roitt I.M., Brostoff J. & Male D. (1985) *Immunology*. Gower Medical Publishing, London

Taussig M.J. (1984) *Processes in Pathology*, 2nd edition. Blackwell Scientific Publications, Oxford.

Major textbooks of haematology (see Chapter 1).

Chapter 7
The leukaemias

The leukaemias are a group of disorders characterised by the accumulation of abnormal white cells in the bone marrow. These abnormal cells may cause bone marrow failure, a raised circulating white cell count and infiltrate other organs. Thus common but not essential features include abnormal white cells in the peripheral blood, a raised total white cell count, evidence of bone marrow failure (i.e. anaemia, neutropenia, thrombocytopenia); and involvement of other organs (e.g. liver, spleen, lymph nodes, meninges, brain, skin, or testis).

Aetiology

The aetiology of leukaemia is unknown. It may result from the interaction of a number of factors.

1 *Neoplasia.* There are obvious similarities between leukaemia and other neoplastic diseases, e.g. uncontrolled proliferation of cells, cellular morphological abnormalities, and organ infiltration. Moreover, other chronic marrow disorders may transform terminally into acute leukaemia, e.g. polycythaemia vera, myelosclerosis or aplastic anaemia. Leukaemia appears to represent a clonal expansion arising by somatic mutation of a single marrow, peripheral lymphoid or thymic cell as shown by chromosomal, isoenzyme, immunological and in-vitro culture techniques. The leukaemia may subsequently develop subclones by the development of new abnormalities and one or more of these subclones may outgrow and replace the initial clone, as shown by the change of chronic granulocytic leukaemia (CGL) from a chronic phase to an acute phase. Usually the subclones are more malignant and often there are new chromosome (cytogenetic) abnormalities.

2 *Infection.* Leukaemia in the mouse and fowl may be transmitted by cell-free filtrates. Virus particles may be demonstrated by electronmicroscopy. In humans, there is now strong evidence for a virus aetiology both in one type of T-cell leukaemia/lymphoma and in Burkitt's lymphoma. The human T leukaemia virus (HTLV), a type c RNA retrovirus, has been demonstrated by

electromicroscopy and by culture in the cells of patients with a particular type of T-cell leukaemia/lymphoma which is common in certain provinces of Japan and which occurs sporadically elsewhere, particularly among Negroes of the Caribbean and United States (p. 171). Epstein-Barr virus, a DNA virus, has been cultured from Burkitt lymphoma tissue and, in this case, the disease is thought to arise because of EB infection in subjects with impaired T-cell immunoregulation, probably due to chronic malaria.

Indirect evidence for a virus aetiology of some leukaemias, is the recurrence of leukaemia in cells of donor origin in about six cases following bone marrow transplantation for acute leukaemia.

3   *Radiation.* Radiation, particularly of the bone marrow, is leukaemogenic. There is an increased incidence of leukaemia in the atomic bomb survivors in Japan, in patients with ankylosing spondylitis who have received spinal irradiation and in children whose mothers received abdominal X-rays during pregnancy.

4   *Hereditary.* There are reports of several cases occurring in one family and in identical twins. Moreover, there is a greatly increased incidence of leukaemia in some hereditary diseases, particularly Down's syndrome (where leukaemia occurs with a 20–30 fold increased frequency), Fanconi anaemia, Bloom's syndrome and ataxia-telangiectasia.

5   *Chemicals.* Chronic exposure to benzene, which may cause bone marrow dysplasia and chromosome changes, is an unusual cause of leukaemia. Other industrial solvents and chemical agents may cause leukaemia less commonly but it is difficult to prove this in an individual case. Chemotherapeutic agents are well established causes, particularly the alkylating drugs such as chlorambucil, mustine and melphalan, and procarbazine. Leukaemia, particularly AML of the myelomonocytic (M_4) and erythroleukaemic (M_6) varieties, is particularly common in patients with lymphomas treated both by radiation and with these drugs.

6   *Chromosome changes* (p. 126).

Classification of leukaemia (Table 7.1)

The main classification is into acute and chronic leukaemia. Acute leukaemia, in which there are over 50% myeloblasts or lymphoblasts in the bone marrow at clinical presentation, is further subdivided into acute myeloid (myeloblastic) leukaemia (AML) and acute lymphoblastic leukaemia (ALL). AML is generally further subdivided into six variants according to the French-American-British (FAB) scheme (Table 7.1). Their treatment and prognosis are basically similar but there are some clinical differences; for example, the M_3 type is associated with disseminated intravascular coagulation (DIC), while the M_4 and M_5 types tend to cause tissue deposits and meningeal leukaemia more frequently than the other

Table 7.1 Classification of leukaemia.

Acute	Chronic
Myeloid (myeloblastic) (AML) Variants	*Chronic granulocytic (CGL)* *Chronic lymphocytic (CLL)*
*M$_1$ myeloblastic poorly differentiated M$_2$ myeloblastic well differentiated M$_3$ promyelocytic M$_4$ myelomonocytic M$_5$ monocytic M$_6$ erythroleukaemia *Megakaryoblastic (rare)* *Lymphoblastic (ALL)* Variants Common ALL (non-T, non-B, cALL antigen positive) null-ALL, non-T non-B Thy-ALL B-cell ALL	Unusual types *Hairy-cell leukaemia* *Prolymphocytic* *Myelodyspastic syndromes* (see p. 150) Also classified as L1, L2, L3 (see below)

* M$_1$–M$_6$ refer to a recently devised (FAB) classification system.

(margin annotations:) DIC. — gum Hyperplasia

variants. Rare cases, presenting with the syndrome of acute myelosclerosis are thought to be of megakaryoblastic origin (see p. 193).

ALL is subdivided according to the FAB classification into L$_1$, L$_2$ and L$_3$ types. These differ in the appearance of the blasts: the L$_1$ type show uniform, smaller cells with less cytoplasm; the L$_2$ type comprise larger cells with more prominent nucleoli and cytoplasm and with more heterogeneity; the L$_3$ type shows cytoplasmic vacuoles. ALL is also subdivided according to immunological markers into common (c), non-T, non-B ALL, which shows the common ALL (cALL) antigen, a null type which is also non-T, non-B but does not show c-ALL antigen, Thy-ALL and B-ALL. B-ALL corresponds usually to the L$_3$ type whereas L$_1$ and L$_2$ types may both be of either c-, null- or Thy-types.

The chronic leukaemias comprise two main types, chronic granulocytic (myeloid) leukaemia (CGL) and chronic lymphocytic (lymphatic) leukaemia (CLL). Other chronic types include hairy cell leukaemia (leukaemic reticulo-endotheliosis), prolymphocytic leukaemia and a variety of myelodysplastic syndromes, some of which are regarded as chronic forms of leukaemia and others as 'pre-leukaemia' (see p. 150).

Cells of origin of the leukaemias and lymphomas

There is now considerable evidence based on similarities of immunological surface membrane phenotype and intracellular en-

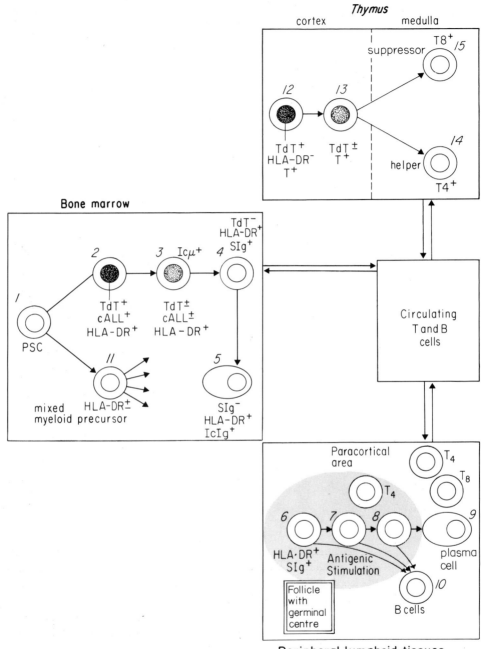

Fig. 7.1 Simplified diagram to show possible cells of origin in the bone marrow, thymus and peripheral lymphoid tissues of the leukaemias, lymphomas and myeloma.

Normal cell	*Suggested tumour derived*
Bone marrow	
1. Pluripotential stem cell	Chronic granulocytic leukaemia
2. Lymphoid progenitor	cALL
3. Pre-B cell	pre-B-ALL
4. B cell	B-ALL
5. Plasma cell	Multiple myeloma
11. Mixed myeloid precursors	AML
Peripheral B-cells (SIg^+, $HLA-DR^+$)	
6. 'Virgin' peripheral B cells ⎫	
7. Follicular peripheral B cell ⎬	CLL, B cell lymphomas
(centrocytic, centroblastic, etc.) ⎭	
8. Lymphoplasmacytoid cells	Macroglobulinaemia
9. Peripheral plasma cell	Peripheral plasmacytoma
10. Coronal lymphocyte	B-prolymphocytic leukaemia
Thymus and T lineage	
12. Large thymic cortical blast ⎫	Thy-ALL, some T lymphomas
13. Thymic cortical cell ⎬	
14. T4$^+$ cell ⎫	Some T lymphomas, mycosis
15. T8$^+$ cell ⎬	fungoides, T-prolymphocytic leukaemia and T-CLL (these probably arise in T cells in peripheral lymphoid tissues)

TdT = terminal deoxynucleotidyl transferase, cALL = antigen present on surface of non-T, non-B, lymphoid 'stem' cell, HLA-DR = histocompatibility-DR antigen (see p. 252), Icμ = intracytoplasmic μ heavy chain, SIg = surface immunoglobulin, T = human T-cell surface antigen.

---

zyme patterns that the leukaemias or lymphomas arise by clonal expansion of one or other cell in the marrow, thymus or peripheral lymphoid tissue (Fig. 7.1). The acute leukaemias are associated with a predominance of myeloblasts or lymphoblasts in the marrow. Acute lymphoblastic leukaemia (ALL) is thought to arise usually from early cells in the lymphoid series; the most common form, common (c)-ALL, does not show T- or B-cell markers but probably arises from a population of very early B-lymphoid progenitors which have nuclear TdT, immunoglobulin gene rearrangement, and show surface HLA-DR (Ia) and common (c)-ALL antigens. In some cases these cells have intracytoplasmic immunoglobulin and are termed pre-B cells. About 10–20% of cases of ALL, termed

Thy-ALL, occur especially in boys and arise from early cortical thymocyte cells which also contain TdT but in addition express T-antigens on the surface, but do not express HLA-DR antigens, thus having the phenotype T^+, TdT^+, HLA-DR, $cALL^-$. A rare form of acute leukaemia, B-ALL, arises from a marrow cell TdT^- but expressing surface immunoglobulin (TdT^-, HLA-DR, SIg^+).

Acute myeloblastic leukaemia (AML) probably arises from a myeloid progenitor, committed in varying degrees to the erythroid, granulocytic-monocytic and megakaryocytic lines. Chronic granulocytic (myeloid) leukaemia probably derives from a very early stem cell, capable of entering both the myeloid or lymphoid lineages and, indeed, it may transform into either acute myeloblastic or acute lymphoblastic leukaemia. Chronic lymphocytic leukaemia (CLL), the B-cell lymphomas, some cases of macroglobulinaemia and peripheral plasmacytomas arise from different cells in the peripheral lymphoid organs, whereas multiple myeloma and some cases of macroglobulinaemia arise from more mature B-cells of the marrow. Certain unusual T-cell disorders: Sézary's syndrome, mycosis fungoides and some T-cell lymphomas and the rare T-CLL arise from more mature T-cells, either of the thymus or of the peripheral lymphoid tissues. The malignant cell in Hodgkin's disease phenotypically resembles a rare cell with certain monocytic features present in normal peripheral lymphoid tissue.

The reason why these particular cells are so prone to give rise to malignant clones, and why these clones escape partly or completely from physiological control factors is unclear, nor is it clear why these different cells give rise to leukaemia (or lymphoma) of particular types at different ages, e.g. why c-ALL is most common in children aged about 4, while AML occurs at any age almost with equal incidence, and myeloma and chronic lymphocytic leukaemia are diseases of older subjects.

Chromosome changes

The Philadelphia (Ph¹) chromosome (see p. 141) is found in the leukaemic cells of the majority of patients with chronic granulocytic leukaemia. Various chromosome abnormalities are found in about 50% of cases of acute leukaemia, e.g. the 8:21 translocation seen in many cases with the M_2 variant of AML, and the Ph¹ chromosome found in the cells of 30–40% of adults with ALL but only rarely in the more common childhood form. In B-ALL and the lymphomas, the most common abnormality is translocation to the long (q) arm of chromosome 14—often from chromosome 8 ($t8q-$; $14q+$)—as in cases of Burkitt lymphoma, B-cell non-Hodgkin's lymphoma and myeloma. Many of these translocations involve movement of cellular oncogenes some of which code for regulators of cell growth and so may theoretically lead to their overexpression.

It is of interest that in many hereditary conditions which predispose to leukaemia (e.g. Down's syndrome and Fanconi anaemia), there are chromosome changes. Moreover, radiation and chemicals may cause persistent chromosome abnormalities before leukaemia develops. Some acquired marrow disorders (e.g. myelodysplastic syndromes) may also show chromosome abnormalities before overt acute leukaemia develops.

THE ACUTE LEUKAEMIAS

Pathogenesis

The leukaemic cell population of ALL and many cases of AML probably results from a clonal proliferation by successive divisions from a single abnormal blast cell. The cells fail to differentiate normally but are capable of further divisions. Their accumulation results in replacement of the normal haemopoietic precursor cells of the bone marrow and, ultimately, in bone marrow failure. The clinical condition of the patient can be correlated with the total number of abnormal leukaemic cells in the body (Fig. 7.2).

The disease may be recognised by conventional morphology only when blast cells in the marrow exceed 4% of the cell total. This corresponds to a total cell count in excess of 10^8. The term 'relapse'

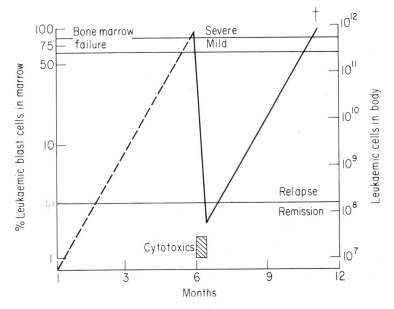

Fig. 7.2 Schematic representation of the pathogenesis of bone marrow failure in acute leukaemia according to the proportion of blast cells in the bone marrow and the mass of leukaemic cells in the body.

is applied to this detectable state. When the number of leukaemic cells is less than 10^8 or 4% of the bone marrow, the leukaemia is usually undetectable by conventional morphology or in 'remission'. When the abnormal cell number approaches 10^{12} the patient is usually gravely ill with severe bone marrow failure. Peripheral blood involvement by the leukaemic cells and infiltration of organs such as the spleen, liver and lymph nodes may not occur until the leukaemic cell population comprises 60% or more of the marrow cell total. The leukaemic cell population in the marrow may be reduced to 'remission' levels by courses of chemotherapy. If no further therapy is given the usual result is a regrowth of leukaemic cells with subsequent haematological and clinical relapse.

The clinical presentation and mortality in acute leukaemia arises mainly from neutropenia, thrombocytopenia and anaemia because of bone marrow failure. In contrast to the chronic leukaemias the total mass of leukaemic tissue at death in untreated patients seldom exceeds 1–2 kg.

Incidence

The acute leukaemias comprise over half of the leukaemias seen in clinical practice. Lymphoblastic leukaemia (ALL) is the common form in children. The incidence is highest at 3–4 years, falling off by ten years. The common type has an equal sex incidence but there is a male predominance for Thy-ALL which also has a later peak age incidence. There is a low frequency after ten years with a secondary rise after the age of 40. Acute myeloid leukaemias occur in all age groups. They are the common form in adults and form only a minor fraction of the leukaemias of childhood.

Clinical features

DUE TO BONE MARROW FAILURE
(i) Pallor, lethargy, dyspnoea from anaemia.
(ii) Fever, malaise, features of mouth, throat, skin, respiratory, perianal or other infections (Fig. 7.3a and 7.3b) including septicaemia are common. The organisms involved are considered in detail below (see p. 132).
(iii) Spontaneous bruises, purpura, bleeding gums and bleeding from venepuncture sites because of thrombocytopenia are common (Fig. 7.3c). Occasionally there is major internal haemorrhage.

DUE TO ORGAN INFILTRATION
(i) Tender bones, especially in children.
(ii) Superficial lymphadenopathy in ALL.
(iii) Moderate splenomegaly, hepatomegaly especially in ALL.
(iv) Gum hypertrophy and infiltration, rectal ulceration, skin in-

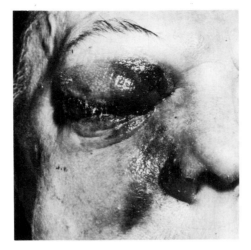

Fig. 7.3a An orbital infection in a female patient (aged 68) with acute myeloblastic leukaemia and severe neutropenia (haemoglobin 8.3 g/dl, white cells 15.3 × 10⁹/l, blasts 96%, neutrophils 1%, platelets 30 × 10⁹/l).

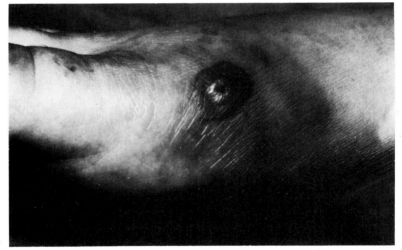

Fig. 7.3b Skin infection (*Pseudomonas pyocyanea*) in a female patient (age 33) with acute lymphoblastic leukaemia receiving chemotherapy and with severe neutropenia (haemoglobin 10.1 g/dl, white cells 0.7 × 10⁹/l, neutrophils 10%, lymphocytes 90%, platelets 20 × 10⁹/l).

volvement (particularly in myelomonocytic, M₄, and monocytic, M₅, types).

(v) Meningeal syndrome (particularly in ALL)—headache, nausea and vomiting, blurring of vision and diplopia. Fundal examination reveals papilloedema and sometimes haemorrhage.

(vi) Other occasional manifestations of organ infiltration include testicular swelling in ALL or signs of mediastinal compression (particularly in Thy-ALL or in the closely related disease of T-lymphoblastic lymphoma (Fig. 7.3d)).

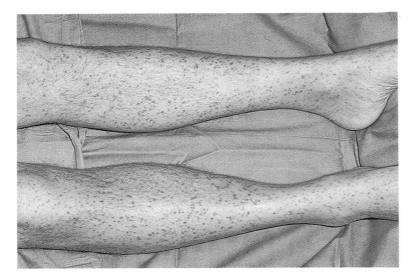

Fig. 7.3c Purpura over the lower limbs in a male patient (age 53) with acute myeloblastic leukaemia (haemoglobin 6.1 g/dl, white cells 20 × 10⁹/1 with 90% blasts, platelets 5 × 10⁹/1).

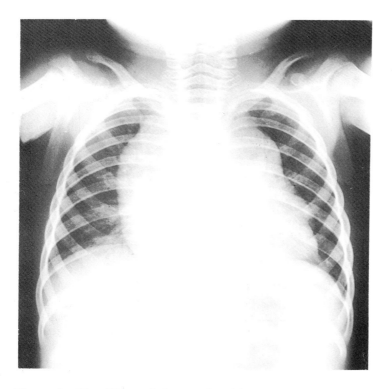

Fig. 7.3d Chest X-ray of a boy aged 6 with Thy-ALL. There is a large mediastinal mass due to thymic enlargement.

Laboratory findings

(i) A normochromic normocytic anaemia.

(ii) The white cell count may be decreased, normal or increased up to $200 \times 10^9/l$ or more.

(iii) Thrombocytopenia in most cases, often extreme in AML.

(iv) Blood film examination typically shows variable numbers of blast cells (Fig. 7.4). In AML, the blasts may contain Auer rods

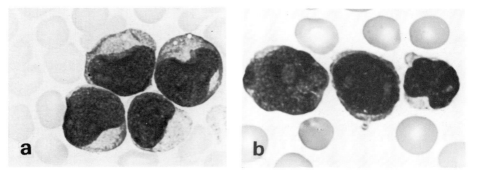

Fig 7.4 Typical blast cells in **a** acute myeloblastic leukaemia (note Auer rod in top left-hand cell), **b** acute lymphoblastic leukaemia.

and other abnormal cells may be present, e.g. promyelocytes, myelocytes, agranular neutrophils, pseudo-Pelger cells, myelomonocytic cells. In erythroleukaemia many erythroblasts are found but these may also be seen in smaller numbers in the other forms. ALL must be differentiated from infectious mononucleosis and other causes of lymphocytosis.

neutrophil alkaline phosphatase.

(v) The bone marrow is hypercellular with a marked proliferation of leukaemic blast cells which typically amount to over 75% of the marrow cell total. In ALL the marrow may be difficult to aspirate because of increased reticulin fibre.

SPECIAL INVESTIGATIONS

Tests for disseminated intravascular coagulation are positive in patients with the promyelocytic (M_3) variant of AML. Lumbar puncture shows that the spinal fluid has an increased pressure and contains leukaemic cells in patients with meningeal leukaemia.

OTHER INVESTIGATIONS

?o

X-rays may reveal lytic bone lesions, expecially in childhood ALL, a mediastinal mass due to enlargement of the thymus and/or mediastinal lymph nodes in Thy-ALL (Fig. 7.3d), infiltration of the lung fields due to infection or less frequently due to the leukaemia itself.

Biochemical tests may reveal a raised serum uric acid and less commonly hypercalcaemia. Liver and renal function tests are performed as a baseline before treatment begins.

DIFFERENTIATION OF ALL AND AML

In most cases, the clinical features and morphology on routine staining separate ALL from AML. In ALL the blasts show no

Table 7.2 Special tests to distinguish ALL blasts from AML blasts (see also Table 7.3).

	ALL	AML
Cytochemistry		
Myeloperoxidase	−	+ (including Auer rods)
Sudan Black	−	+
Non-specific esterase	−	+ in monocytic types
Periodic Schiff (PAS)	+ (coarse)	+ (fine)
Acid phosphatase	+ in Thy-ALL	
Enzyme test		
Terminal deoxynucleotidyl transferase (TdT)	+	−
Serum lysozyme	−	+ + in monocytic types
Electronmicroscopy	−	+ (early granule formation)
Gene rearrangements	rearrangement of immunoglobulin genes (c-ALL) or T-cell receptor (Thy-ALL)	germline configuration of immunoglobulin genes and T cell receptor genes

Table 7.3 Immunological markers useful for subdividing leukaemia.

	c-ALL (non-T, non-B ALL)	Thy-ALL	B-ALL, CLL, other mature B-cell tumours	AML
anti-c-ALL	+	−	−	−
anti-HLA-DR	+	−	+	±
anti-TdT	+	+	−	−
E-ros	−	+	−	−
anti-Thy	−	+	−	−
SIg	−	−	+	−

c-ALL = common-ALL antigen; HLA-DR (see p. 256); TdT = terminal deoxynucleotidyl transferase; Thy = thymic antigen; E-ros = rosettes with sheep red cells; SIg = surface immunoglobulin. null-ALL resembles c-ALL but c-ALL antigen is absent.

differentiation whereas in AML some evidence of differentiation to granulocytes is usually seen in the blasts or their progeny. Special tests are needed when the cells are undifferentiated and to sub-divide cases of ALL into its different types.

Cytochemistry. This may help to show granule development in myeloblastic disorders and distinguish other cell types (Table 7.2).

Immunological markers and enzyme assays. These are particularly helpful in sub-dividing ALL into the common (non-B, non-T) variety (c-ALL), null-ALL, Thy-ALL (thymic cell origin) and the rare B-ALL. They also help to differentiate ALL from AML. The enzyme TdT (Table 7.3), which is raised in ALL and normal in AML blasts, may also be detected biochemically or immunologically and is a useful marker. Detection of rearrangement of immunoglobulin genes (pp. 118–9) or T-cell receptor genes is a new sensitive method for detecting a monoclonal population of early B-cells (as c-ALL or B-ALL) or T-cells (as in Thy-ALL).

Management: Supportive care

General supportive therapy for bone marrow failure includes the following:

INSERTION OF A CENTRAL VENOUS CATHETER: it is usual to insert a central venous catheter (e.g. Hickman) via a skin tunnel from the chest into the superior vena cava to give ease of access for blood, blood products, antibiotics, intravenous feeding, etc. and for blood sampling for laboratory tests.

TREATMENT OF ANAEMIA: red cell transfusions.

TREATMENT AND PROPHYLAXIS OF HAEMORRHAGE: platelet concentrates and fresh blood are used. As haemorrhage is an important cause of death soon after presentation, regular platelet concentrates are given in the management of patients with repeated minor haemorrhage and in all cases with severe thrombocytopenia (platelets less than $20 \times 10^9/l$) and during the initial induction therapy when severe thrombocytopenia is likely. Replacement of clotting factors with fresh frozen plasma and platelet transfusions are needed particularly in patients with DIC due to the M_3 variant of AML before and during initial chemotherapy.

TREATMENT AND PROPHYLAXIS OF INFECTION

Types of infection

Neutropenia due to bone marrow replacement by leukaemic blasts and because of intensive cytotoxic therapy renders the patient exquisitely susceptible to infection, particularly when the absolute neutrophil count falls below $0.5 \times 10^9/l$. In many patients, neutrophil counts of $0.2 \times 10^9/l$ or less persist for several weeks. The infections are predominantly bacterial and usually arise from the patient's own commensal bacterial flora — most commonly Gram-negative gut bacteria, e.g. *Pseudomonas pyocyanea*, *E. coli*, *Proteus*, *Klebsiella* and anaerobes. Staphylococcal and streptococcal infections are also frequent and organisms not normally considered pathogenic, e.g. *Staphylococcus epidermidis*, may cause life-threatening infection. Moreover, in the absence of neutrophils, local superficial lesions rapidly cause severe septicaemia. Viral (e.g. *Herpes simplex* and *zoster*), fungal (e.g. *Candida*), and protozoal (e.g. *Pneumocystis carinii*) infections also occur with increased frequency, particularly when neutropenia is prolonged and multiple courses of antibiotics have been used to treat possible bacterial infection. The following measures help to deal with this dominant problem of susceptibility to infection.

Prophylaxis of infection

Isolation facilities. Patients should be nursed in separate rooms preferably with 'reverse-barrier' isolation techniques or placed in 'laminar air-flow' rooms.

Reduction of gut and other commensal flora. Bowel sterilisation with FRAmycetin, COlistin and Nystatin (FRACON) or other regimens of non-absorbed antibiotics and antifungal agents (e.g. ketoconazole or amphotericin) is used by many units. Prophylactic co-trimoxazole has also been shown to be effective. Regular cultures should be taken from urine, faeces, sputum, vagina, throat, gums, nose, drip sites, axillary, umbilical and perineal skin areas to document the patient's bacterial flora and its sensitivity. Topical antiseptics are used for bathing and for treating any site where pathogens are detected. If these are not eliminated, systemic antibiotic therapy is considered.

Treatment of infection

Fever is an excellent indicator that infection is present. Blood cultures and cultures from any likely focus should be taken immediately fever occurs and vigorous attempts made to identify the responsible organism by direct examination of possibly infected material as well as by culture methods. The mouth and throat, drip sites, the perineal and perianal areas are particularly likely foci. Because of the absence of neutrophils, pus is not formed and infections are not localised. The absence of a neutrophil reaction makes the severity of infections of, for example, the lungs, urine, or skin more difficult to assess. Chest X-ray and urine culture are essential. Antibiotic therapy must be started immediately. In at least half the febrile episodes no organisms are isolated. An aminoglycoside (e.g. gentamicin or netilmicin) in combination with a penicillin active against pseudomonas (e.g. mezlocillin, ticarcillin or piperacillin) or with a cephalosporin in high dosage has been proved an excellent initial combination. These cover Gram-negative organisms including pseudomonas as well as Gram-positive cocci and are effective bactericidal drugs despite severe neutropenia. As soon as the infective agent and its antibiotic sensitivity are known appropriate changes in the regimen must be made. If no response occurs, the possibility of anaerobic organisms, fungal or viral infections, should be considered and appropriate therapy given, e.g. with metronidazole, antifungal or antiviral drugs. Acyclovir has been shown to be an effective agent against herpes infection. These infections are most likely to occur after initial infective episodes have been treated but bone marrow recovery has not occurred.

Leucocyte concentrates prepared on cell separators from normal donors or patients with chronic granulocytic leukaemia are given to severely neutropenic patients with life-threatening septicaemias or extensive local infections not responding within 24–48 hours to antibiotics.

Management: Cytotoxic drug therapy

Most of the cytotoxic drugs used in leukaemia therapy damage the capacity of the cell for reproduction (Table 7.4). Combinations of at least three drugs are now usually used initially to increase the cytotoxic effect, improve remission rates and reduce the frequency of emergence of drug resistance. These multiple drug combinations have also been found to give longer remissions than single agents.

Initial therapy may be accompanied by hyperkalaemia and hyperuricaemia and uric acid nephropathy, and thus the patient should be given allopurinol before starting therapy and well hydrated.

The aim of cytotoxic therapy is firstly to induce a remission (absence of any clinical or laboratory evidence of the disease) and then continually to reduce the hidden leukaemic cell population by repeated courses of therapy. Cyclical combinations of two, three or four drugs are given with treatment-free intervals to allow the bone marrow to recover (Fig. 7.5). This recovery depends upon the differential regrowth pattern of normal haemopoietic and leukaemic cells.

Cytotoxic therapy of acute lymphoblastic leukaemia

Prednisolone, vincristine and asparaginase are the drugs usually used to achieve remission in over 90% of children in 4–6 weeks. Daunorubicin or hydroxodaunorubicin (Adriamycin) is added to the regimen either in the induction phase or in consolidation once remission has been achieved (Fig. 7.6).

The following groups carry a less favourable prognosis:
1 Males compared to females.
2 Those with an initial high leucocyte count (e.g. $> 20 \times 10^9/l$).

Table 7.4 Drugs used in the treatment of leukaemia.

	Mechanism of action	Particular side-effects*
Antimetabolites		
Methotrexate	Inhibit pyrimidine or purine synthesis or incorporation into DNA	Mouth ulcers, gut toxicity
6-Mercaptopurine		
6-Thioguanine		Jaundice
Cytosine arabinoside		Gut toxicity, haemolytic anaemia
Hydroxyurea		Gut toxicity, skin atrophy
Alkylating agents		
Cyclophosphamide	Cross-link DNA, impede RNA formation	Haemorrhagic cystitis, cardiomyopathy, loss of hair
Chlorambucil		Marrow aplasia, hepatic toxicity, dermatitis
Busulphan (Myleran)		Marrow aplasia, pulmonary fibrosis, hyper-pigmentation
DNA binding		
Daunorubicin Hydroxodaunorubi-cin (Adriamycin)	Bind to DNA and interfere with mitosis	Cardiac toxicity, hair loss
Mitotic inhibitor		
Vincristine (Oncovin)	Spindle damage, absent metaphase	Neuropathy (peripheral or bladder or gut), hair loss
Miscellaneous		
Corticosteroids	Uncertain	Peptic ulcer, obesity, diabetes, osteoporosis, psychosis
L-Asparaginase	Deprive cells of asparagine	Hypersensitivity, low albumin and coagulation factors, pancreatitis
Epipodophyllotoxin (VP16-213)	Mitotic inhibitor	Alopecia, oral ulceration

* Most of the drugs cause nausea, vomiting and bone marrow toxicity.

3 Very young (< 2 years) or older patients (adolescents or adults).
4 Patients who have meningeal involvement at presentation.
5 Thy-cell leukaemia (20% of all cases) or the rare B-ALL.
   In these cases, treatment with a more intensive induction regi-

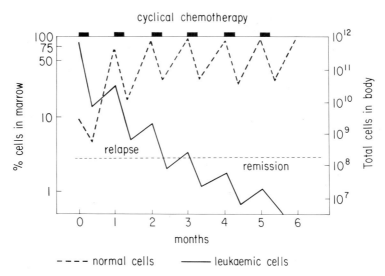

Fig. 7.5 The effect of cyclic therapy on the blast cells and normal haemopoietic cells in acute leukaemia.

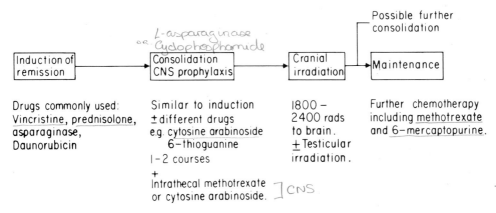

L-asparaginase
or Cyclophosphamide

| Induction of remission | Consolidation CNS prophylaxis | Cranial irradiation | Maintenance |

Possible further consolidation

Drugs commonly used:
Vincristine, prednisolone,
asparaginase,
Daunorubicin

Similar to induction
±different drugs
e.g. cytosine arabinoside
6-thioguanine
1-2 courses
+
Intrathecal methotrexate
or cytosine arabinoside.] CNS

1800 –
2400 rads
to brain.
± Testicular
irradiation.

Further chemotherapy
including methotrexate
and 6-mercaptopurine.

Fig. 7.6 A flow chart for a typical treatment regimen for acute lymphoblastic leukaemia.

men is used; although predisposing to early complications, this improves the chances of long-term survival.

Overall, between 30 and 50% of children with common ALL (non-T, non-B) are now alive and off all treatment five years from their presentation. It seems likely that many of them are cured. In other patients, death occurs during initial treatment or subsequent maintenance therapy, or during re-induction after relapse, usually from infection due to neutropenia and immunosuppression. Relapsed disease is more difficult to treat and second remissions, if obtained, are usually of short duration. Thy-ALL is particularly likely to relapse.

Leukaemic cells in the meninges are beyond the reach of most of the cytotoxic drugs used in therapy. Meningeal leukaemia used to occur in three of every four children during the first four years after diagnosis of ALL. Repopulation of the bone marrow from the meninges results in haematological relapse.

Cranial irradiation (1800–2400 rads) and courses of intrathecal methotrexate during initial treatment and after the remission has been obtained are now used in all cases of ALL under 40 years old to prevent CNS relapse. A significant improvement in the rate of survival occurs. CNS relapse may still occur and presents with headache, vomiting, papilloedema and blast cells in the CSF. It is treated with intrathecal methotrexate (or cytosine arabinoside). In children less than two years old, irradiation is better avoided.

Testicular relapse may occur in boys and prophylactic testicular irradiation appears to provide some benefit in survival, although it renders the patient permanently sterile.

MAINTENANCE CHEMOTHERAPY

This is given for 2–3 years normally, with daily mercaptopurine and weekly methotrexate. More complicated regimens exist with vincristine, steroids and other drugs added. Trials of intensive early or later chemotherapeutic consolidation regimens are also in progress in poor risk cases.

There is a high risk of varicella or measles during therapy in children who lack immunity to these viruses. If exposure to these infections occurs, prophylactic immunoglobulin should be given.

Cytotoxic therapy of acute myeloblastic leukaemia

The therapeutic attack on AML is similar to that described for ALL but the results are less good. The most commonly used regimen for AML is a combination of the three drugs cytosine arabinoside, daunorubicin and 6-thioguanine (Fig. 7.7). Cases of

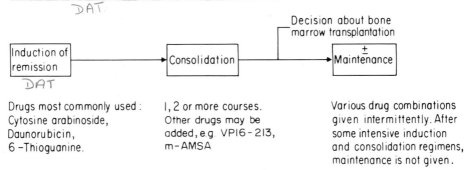

Fig. 7.7 A flow chart for a typical treatment regimen for acute myeloblastic leukaemia.

all the AML subtypes (FAB M_1–M_6) are treated similarly (except that disseminated intravascular coagulation is likely in the promyelocytic (M_3) variant and platelet concentrates and fresh frozen plasma to provide clotting factors are used until remission is obtained). A typical good response is shown in Fig. 7.8. Compared with ALL:

1 The remission rate is lower (60–80%).

2 Remission often takes longer to achieve.

3 Only myelotoxic drugs are of major value, with less selectivity between leukaemic and normal marrow cells.

4 Marrow failure is severe and prolonged, intensive supportive care is required and early deaths are common, particularly in patients over 50.

5 Remissions are shorter, the value of maintenance therapy is less obvious, and long-term survivors are unusual.

CNS prophylaxis is not usually given in AML, although meningeal relapse does occur in some cases, especially children and young adults, in whom intrathecal methotrexate may be used prophylactically.

In a number of older patients presenting with variants of AML the disease runs a 'smouldering' or subacute course. These patients may have enough platelets and neutrophils initially to prevent life-threatening haemorrhage or infection but they respond poorly to aggressive anti-leukaemic therapy. Supportive transfusions and the judicious use of mild chemotherapy are often the best form of treatment in these cases, as long as blasts form less than 50% of the marrow population.

Bone marrow transplantation

Allogeneic (HLA and mixed lymphocyte culture, compatible sibling) bone marrow transplantation is now being used in some centres in patients under 45 years old with AML in first remission, and in ALL patients who relapse and achieve a successful second remission after re-induction cytotoxic therapy. It is also considered in some ALL patients in first remission with a particularly poor prognosis (e.g. a white count of $> 100 \times 10^9/l$ at presentation). Transplantation is performed to reconstitute the patient's haemopoietic system after total body irradiation and intensive chemotherapy is given in attempts to kill all remaining leukaemic cells. The preliminary results of these trials are encouraging with perhaps 50% long-term survivors. If a syngeneic donor (identical twin) is available, bone marrow transplantation should be carried out both in ALL and AML at the time of the first remission.

Prognosis of acute leukaemia

The prognosis of ALL in children has been improved greatly by

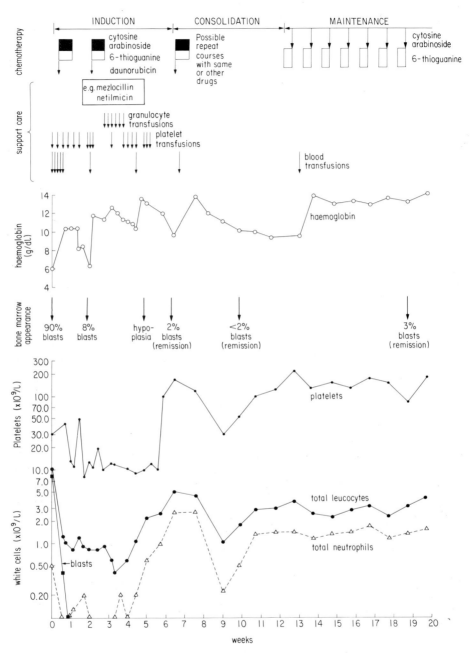

Fig. 7.8 A haematological chart of the treatment of a patient (female age 22) with acute myeloblastic leukaemia. The chart is used to monitor the patient's response to chemotherapy and to record the support therapy). Various drug regimens are used and that given here is one example.

Table 7.5 Prognosis in treated acute leukaemia.

	Median survival (months)
ALL (children)	
without CNS prophylaxis	33.0
with CNS prophylaxis	60.0 +
ALL (adults)	12.0–18.0
AML	12.0–18.0

Note   The median survival of all patients with acute leukaemia in 1948 was 2.0 months.

the use of chemotherapy, radiotherapy, better supportive therapy and the development of special leukaemia units. Progress in AML has been less spectacular. The approximate median survival figures are shown in Table 7.5.

CHRONIC GRANULOCYTIC (MYELOID) LEUKAEMIA

Chronic granulocytic (myeloid, myelogenous) leukaemia comprises 20% of all the leukaemias and is seen most frequently in middle age. In over 90% of patients there is a replacement of normal bone marrow by cells with an abnormal G group chromosome (no. 22)— the Philadelphia or Ph¹ chromosome (Fig. 7.9). This abnormality is a translocation of part of a long (q) arm of chromosome 22 to another chromosome, usually 9 in the 'C' group. It is an acquired abnormality that is present in all dividing granulocytic, erythroid and megakaryocytic cells in the marrow and also in B lymphocytes. A great increase in total body granulocyte mass is responsible for most of the clinical features. In at least 70% of patients there is a terminal metamorphosis to an acute malignant form of leukaemia.

Clinical features

This disease occurs in either sex, most frequently between the ages of 50 and 60; however, it may occur even in childhood. Its clinical features include the following:

(i) Symptoms related to hypermetabolism, e.g. weight loss, lassitude, anorexia, night sweats.

(ii) Splenomegaly is nearly always present and is frequently massive. In some patients this enlargement is associated with considerable discomfort, pain or indigestion.

(iii) Features of anaemia may include pallor, dyspnoea and tachycardia.

(iv) Bruising, epistaxis, menorrhagia or haemorrhage from other sites.

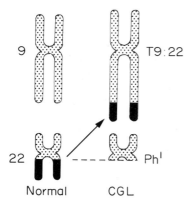

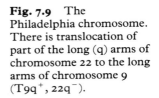

Fig. 7.9 The Philadelphia chromosome. There is translocation of part of the long (q) arms of chromosome 22 to the long arms of chromosome 9 (T9q$^+$, 22q$^-$).

(v) Less common features include gout, visual disturbance and other neurological symptoms, priapism.

(vi) Occasional patients are detected during routine blood examination.

Laboratory investigations

DIAGNOSTIC FEATURES

(i) Leucocytosis usually $> 50 \times 10^9$/l and sometimes $> 500 \times 10^9$/l.

(ii) A complete spectrum of myeloid cells is seen in the peripheral blood. The levels of neutrophils and myelocytes exceed those of blast cells and promyelocytes (Fig. 7.10).

ADDITIONAL FEATURES

(i) Philadelphia chromosome on cytogenetic analysis of blood or bone marrow.

(ii) Bone marrow is hypercellular with granulopoietic predominance.

(iii) Neutrophil alkaline phosphatase score invariably low. ⚹.

(iv) Increased circulating basophils.

(v) Normochromic, normocytic anaemia is usual.

(vi) Platelet count may be increased, normal or decreased.

(vii) Serum vitamin B_{12} and vitamin B_{12}-binding capacity are increased.

Treatment

There is a predictable response to therapy in the chronic phase. By reducing the total granulocyte mass, cytotoxic drugs are able to keep patients symptom free for long periods.

Busulphan. This alkylating agent is the treatment of choice. Regular blood counts allow the dose to be titrated in individual patients (Fig. 7.11). Some regimens employ 6-mercaptopurine or 6-thio-

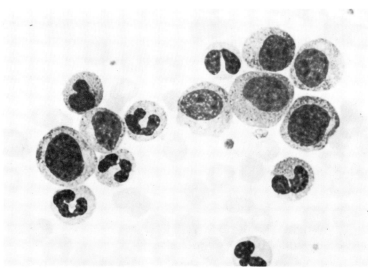

Fig. 7.10 Peripheral blood film from a patient (male age 45) with chronic granulocytic leukaemia showing myelocytes, metamyelocytes and mature neutrophils. Blood count: haemoglobin 10.6 g/dl, white cells $250 \times 10^9/l$, platelets $500 \times 10^9/l$.

guanine in combination with busulphan or use busulphan in intermittent high doses rather than in daily lower doses.

Dibromomannitol, Hydroxyurea. These are useful alternatives for occasional patients who are resistant to or having side-effects from busulphan.

Allopurinol. This prevents high urate production with consequent gout or renal damage.

Splenic irradiation or splenectomy are usually reserved for patients whose splenic enlargement is not responsive to chemotherapy. Elective splenectomy is recommended in some centres but is of no proven value.

Bone marrow transplantation. Allogenic bone marrow transplantation in the initial phase is probably the best treatment for patients of 50 or younger, who have an HLA-, MLC-matched sibling. This is the only treatment regularly leading to elimination of the Ph¹ positive clone of cells and offering a strong chance of permanent cure.

COURSE AND PROGNOSIS

CGL has a very constant clinical course with an excellent response to chemotherapy in the chronic phase. The median survival is 3–4 years. Death usually occurs from terminal acute transformation

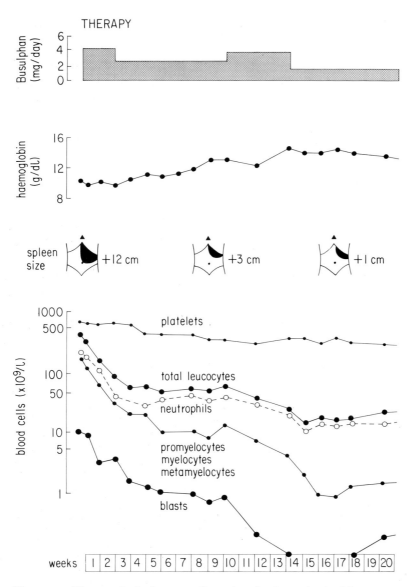

Fig. 7.11 Haematological course of a patient (male aged 39) with chronic granulocytic leukaemia initially treated with busulphan.

or from intercurrent haemorrhage or infection. Twenty per cent of patients survive 10 years or more.

Metamorphosis of CGL (blast cell or acute transformation)

The patient becomes refractory to therapy usually with severe anaemia, thrombocytopenia and an increase in blast cells in the blood and marrow. This acute transformation may be in an accelerated phase for several months during which the disease is less easy to control than in the chronic phase. In the acute phase, new chromosome abnormalities are often present. In about one-third of cases the transformation is lymphoblastic and then there may be a temporary response to therapy with vincristine and corticosteroids. Survival beyond transformation is brief, however, and rarely more than twelve months.

Variants of CGL

1 Juvenile CML. A Ph¹-negative variant which occurs in young children, often with extensive lymphadenopathy, and responds poorly to treatment.

Atypical 2 Philadelphia-negative CGL. This variant shows minor haematological differences to Ph¹-positive disease and responds less well to therapy.

3 Eosinophilic leukaemia. This is often difficult to distinguish from the hypereosinophilia syndrome in which hepatosplenomegaly, rashes, cardiac and pulmonary abnormalities occur. In the leukaemia, more blasts are present and cytogenetic abnormalities may also be seen.

4 Chronic myelomonocytic leukaemia (see p. 151).

CHRONIC LYMPHOCYTIC LEUKAEMIA (CLL)

Chronic lymphocytic (lymphatic) leukaemia accounts for 25% of the leukaemias seen in clinical practice and occurs chiefly in the elderly. Although classified as a lymphoproliferative disorder, in most patients there is little evidence of an aggressive proliferation of the abnormal lymphocytes. The accumulation of large numbers of lymphocytes to 50–100 times the normal lymphoid mass in the blood, bone marrow, spleen and liver may be related to immunological non-reactivity and excessive lifespan. In most cases the cells are a monoclonal population of B-lymphocytes but in a few they are all T-cells. With advanced disease there is often bone marrow failure, a tumorous syndrome with generalised discrete lymphadenopathy and sometimes soft tissue lymphoid masses; immunological failure results from reduced humoral and cellular immune processes.

Clinical features

(i) Symmetrical enlargement of superficial lymph nodes is found in most patients (Fig. 7.12a). The nodes are usually discrete and not tender.

(ii) Features of anaemia, e.g. pallor, dyspnoea.

(iii) Splenomegaly and hepatomegaly are usual.

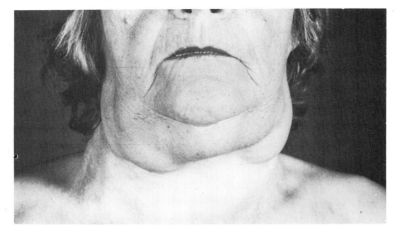

Fig. 7.12a Cervical lymphadenopathy in a patient with chronic lymphocytic leukaemia (female age 73).

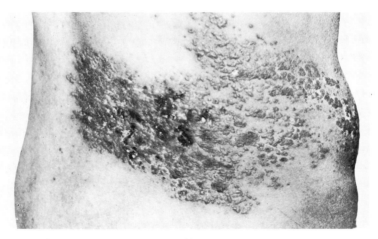

Fig. 7.12b Herpes zoster infection in a patient with chronic lymphocytic leukaemia (female age 68).

(iv) Patients with thrombocytopenia may show bruising or purpura.

(v) Pruritus occurs in many patients, and there is an association with herpes zoster (Fig. 7.12b). In some patients zoster is the initial manifestation. Excessive reactions to vaccination and insect bites also occur. Skin infiltration is present in a small number of patients.

(vi) Tonsillar enlargement may be a feature. Involvement of the salivary and lacrimal glands (Mikulicz's syndrome) is a rare but interesting presentation.

(vii) About 20% of cases are diagnosed when a routine blood test is performed.

Laboratory findings

(i) *Leucocytosis:* The absolute lymphocyte count is above $5 \times 10^9/l$ and, in the majority of patients, is $30–300 \times 10^9/l$. Between 70 and 99% of white cells in the blood film appear as small lymphocytes (Fig. 7.13). Smudge or smear cells are also present.

(ii) Normocytic, normochromic anaemia is present in later stages. Autoimmune haemolysis may also occur (see below).

(iii) Thrombocytopenia occurs in many patients. *Autoimmune Thrombocytic Purpura.*

(iv) Bone marrow aspiration shows lymphocytic replacement of normal marrow elements. Lymphocytes comprise 25–95% of all the cells.

(v) Reduced concentration of serum immunoglobulins are found in most patients, particularly with advanced disease.

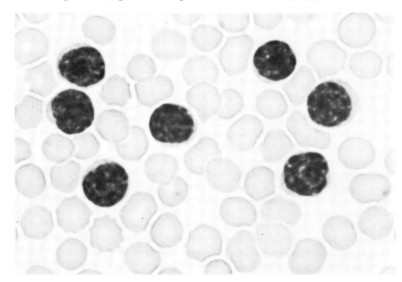

Fig. 7.13 Peripheral blood film in chronic lymphocytic leukaemia (patient illustrated in Fig. 7.12a). Numerous small lymphocytes are present.

Variants of CLL

1 CLL may be asymptomatic, especially in older patients without abnormal physical signs. The course of this benign form may remain stable for many years and these patients often need no treatment.

2 A more aggressive form may be seen in younger patients aged 30–50 where it is characterised by fatigue, weight loss, anorexia, sweating, progressive lymphadenopathy, hepatosplenomegaly, bone marrow and immunological failure.

3 Some 10–15% of CLL patients develop a *secondary autoimmune haemolytic anaemia* associated with jaundice, marked reticulocytosis, spherocytosis and a positive direct Coombs' (antiglobulin) test. A secondary auto-immune thrombocytopenia occurs in about 5% of patients.

4 Prolymphocytic leukaemia is a variant of CLL characterised by massive splenomegaly and lymphocyte counts up to and sometimes exceeding $400 \times 10^9/l$ but absent lymph node enlargement. The response to treatment is poor. The cells are large with a prominent nucleolus and immature nucleus. They are usually B- but T-types also occur.

5 Chronic T-cell leukaemia forms 1% of all cases of CLL and occurs in younger subjects than the usual B-CLL. There is also less lymphadenopathy, more cutaneous involvement, and a poor response to therapy.

Treatment

The disease has been divided into five stages (Rai *et al* (1975) *Blood* **46,** 219) with progressively shorter survival:

    o. Absolute lymphocytosis $> 15 \times 10^9/l$.

    I. As Stage o + enlarged lymph nodes.

    II. As Stage o + enlarged liver and/or spleen*. ± adenopathy.

    III. As Stage o + anaemia (Hb < 11 g/dl)*‡.

    IV. As Stage o + thrombocytopenia (platelets $< 100 \times 10^9/l$)*†‡.

* ± adenopathy

† ± organomegaly

‡ autoimmune haemolytic anaemia or thrombocytopenia do not make the patient stage III or IV.

    There is no need to treat Stage o but patients in the other stages need treatment, particularly if there is: **a** Evidence of bone marrow failure; **b** symptomatic involvement of lymph nodes and skin; **c** splenomegaly causing 'hypersplenism' or symptoms; **d** autoimmune haemolytic anaemia or thrombocytopenia.

Corticosteroids. Patients in bone marrow failure should be treated initially with prednisolone alone until there is significant recovery of the platelet, neutrophil and haemoglobin levels. The peripheral white count initially rises as infiltrated organs shrink, but later the count falls. Corticosteroids are also indicated in autoimmune haemolytic anaemia or thrombocytopenia.

Alkylating agents. Continuous or intermittent therapy with either chlorambucil or cyclophosphamide successfully reduces total lymphocyte mass and may prevent bone marrow failure for periods of several years until the lymphocytes become refractory.

Radiotherapy is useful for treating lymph nodes or local deposits causing pressure symptoms and also for reducing spleen size in patients with hypersplenism.

Splenectomy is indicated for auto-immune haemolytic anaemia which does not respond to steroids and alkylating agents and for occasional patients with massive splenomegaly which is refractory to therapy and causing symptoms of 'hypersplenism'.

Ancillary therapy includes active treatment and prophylaxis of infection with antibacterial and antifungal aspects. Regular injections of gammaglobulin may help patients with severe hypogammaglobulinaemia who are having recurrent infections. Allopurinol reduces urate production in patients with high lymphocyte counts. Supportive transfusions with red cells or platelets may be required for patients in bone marrow failure.

Prognosis

Most patients with CLL live for 3–5 years. Patients with slowly progressive disease or the 'benign' form often survive for ten years (Rai Stage 0, mean survival 12 years or more, while Stage I patients have a mean survival of 8 years). Unlike CGL, CLL does not transform into acute leukaemia. Death is usually due to infection due to bone marrow failure and immune deficiency.

HAIRY-CELL LEUKAEMIA

This is an unusual disease of peak age 40–60 with a male to female ratio of 4 : 1; it is characterised clinically by features due to pancytopenia. The spleen may be moderately enlarged. There is a monoclonal proliferation of cells with an irregular cytoplasmic outline ('hairy' cells, a type of B-lymphocyte) in the peripheral blood, bone marrow, liver and other organs. The bone marrow trephine shows a characteristic appearance of mild fibrosis and a diffuse cellular infiltrate. A serum paraprotein may be present. Splenectomy may improve the haematological picture if the spleen is large. Excellent haematological responses and complete remission of the *some cases* disease have recently been described with prolonged therapy with interferon. The course is often chronic, requiring only supportive therapy with an overall mean survival of 4–5 years—though some patients live very much longer.

LYMPHOSARCOMA CELL LEUKAEMIA

This is normally associated with B-cell tumours of the follicle centre cell type (with indented or cleaved nuclei) and the course is that of a non-Hodgkin's lymphoma (p. 162). The blood film shows abnormal lymphoid cells.

SEZARY SYNDROME

This is a leukaemic variant of mycoses fungoides (see p. 171).

MYELODYSPLASTIC SYNDROMES

In these conditions, qualitative and quantitative abnormalities occur in one or more of the three myeloid cell lines: red cells, granulocytes and monocytes, and platelets. The clinical course is characterised by anaemia, infections due to impaired phagocytic production and/or function and haemorrhage due to thrombocytopenia or impaired platelet function. These syndromes occur in either sex and most commonly in middle or old age. A wide spectrum of peripheral blood and bone marrow abnormalities may occur with macrocytosis, ring sideroblasts, megaloblastic erythropoiesis, disordered granulopoiesis and megakaryocytes, and chromosome abnormalities.

The FAB classification (Table 7.6) includes cases of primary acquired sideroblastic anaemia and refractory anaemia without excess blasts in this spectrum of diseases. Others would regard primary acquired sideroblastic anaemia as a relatively benign and separate somatic mutation of the bone marrow (see p. 40) and classify 'refractory anaemia without excess blasts' as one type of 'pre-leukaemia'. The term 'smouldering' leukaemia has been used to describe variants of these syndromes which are more clearly leukaemic. Ultimately, after months or years of follow-up, a variable proportion of all types transforms into acute myeloblastic leukaemia which proves fatal.

Table 7.6 The French-American-British (FAB) classification of the myelodysplastic syndrome (Bennett *et al* (1982) *British Journal of Haematology* **51**, 189–99).

1	Refractory anaemia (RA)*
2	RA with ring sideroblasts (ring sideroblasts $> 15\%$)
3	RA with excess blasts (RAEB) (blasts 5–20%)
4	Chronic myelomonocytic leukaemia (CMML)
5	RAEB 'in transformation' (blasts 20–30%)

* Some cases of neutropenia or thrombocytopenia, with or without anaemia, are included in this category ('refractory cytopenia'). See also 'pre-leukaemia', p. 151.

t.o.c Retinoic Acid — helps cells not differentiating v. quickly to ↑ Rate of "

Chronic myelomonocytic leukaemia (CMML)

In this syndrome, the blood picture may resemble that of CGL except the total leucocyte count is lower and the absolute monocyte count is raised and Ph[1] chromosome is absent. There are increases in the proportion of monocytes in the blood and myeloblasts in the bone marrow; abnormal granulocytes may be seen in the peripheral blood and marrow, e.g. agranular, pseudo-Pelger cells or cells intermediate between granulocytes and monocytes. The platelet count and absolute neutrophil count may be low. Neutrophil or platelet dysfunction also occur and may account for infections or bleeding in the face of normal numbers of neutrophils or platelets in some patients. Anaemia of a varying degree is usual and ring sideroblasts are present in the marrow. Treatment is with supportive therapy alone or with mild chemotherapy (e.g. 6-mercaptopurine) until acute myeloblastic transformation occurs.

Refractory anaemia with excess blasts (RAEB)

The clinical course of patients with this syndrome resembles that of chronic myelomonocytic leukaemia except anaemia is usually more marked and monocytosis is absent. The bone marrow shows 5-20% blasts. The anaemia is often macrocytic and abnormal precursors including ring sideroblasts may occur in the bone marrow. Morphological and functional abnormalities of the neutrophils and platelets are usual and their marrow precursors are abnormal. Treatment is supportive, sometimes with mild chemotherapy, e.g. low dose cytosine arabinoside. Aggressive treatment is usually withheld until the proportion of blasts in the bone marrow is over 30%, although some would treat accelerated phase RAEB with 20-30% blasts, particularly if the patient has severe infections or bleeding problems, with AML-type therapy.

Pre-leukaemia

This is an ill-defined diagnosis made on a number of chronic acquired bone marrow abnormalities which, in a proportion of patients, progress to leukaemia—usually of the acute myeloblastic variety. Most haematologists reserve this term for patients with a refractory anaemia and/or neutropenia or thrombocytopenia, macrocytosis and megaloblastic bone marrow not responding to vitamin B_{12} or folic acid. There is often disordered granulopoiesis and megakaryocytes and abnormalities of chromosomes and bone marrow culture pattern in semi-solid agar. The proportion of blasts in the marrow is less than 5%. This type of 'pre-leukaemia' corresponds closely to refractory anaemia (cytopenia) in the FAB classification (FAB_1) (see Table 7.6). Some patients with acquired sideroblastic anaemia, aplastic anaemia, red cell aplasia, and a variety of mild 'dysmyelopoietic syndromes' ultimately develop acute leukaemia

leukaemia and the prodromal phase could then be termed, in retro-spect, pre-leukaemia. Other cases with very similar initial blood and bone marrow abnormalities do not progress to definite leu-kaemia even after many years of follow-up. Because of this many clinicians prefer not to use the term pre-leukaemia at all.

SELECTED BIBLIOGRAPHY

Catovsky D. (ed.) (1981) *The Leukaemic Cell*. Churchill-Livingstone, Edinburgh.

Chaganti R.S.K. (1983) Significance of chromosome changes to hematopoietic neoplasms. *Blood* **62,** 515.

Clinics in Hematology (1982) vol. 11.3, *The lymphocytes*. Ed. G. Janossy. W.B. Saunders, Philadelphia.

Clinics in Haematology (1984) vol. 13.2, *Infections and Leukaemia*. Ed. H.G. Prentice. W.B. Saunders, Philadelphia.

Clinics in Haematology (1977) vol. 6.1, *The Chronic Leukaemias*. Ed. D.A.G. Galton. W.B. Saunders, Philadelphia.

Clinics in Haematology (1980) vol 9.1, *Cytogenics and Haematology*. Ed. D.G. Pennington. W.B. Saunders, Philadelphia.

Gale R.P. (ed.) (1983) *Recent Advances in Bone Marrow Transplantation*, Alan R. Liss, New York.

Galton D.A.G. (1981) Chronic Leukaemia. In *Recent Advances in Haematology 3*, ed. A.V. Hoffbrand. Churchill-Livingstone, Edinburgh.

Gunz F.W. & Henderson E.S. (1983) *Leukaemia*, 4th edition. Grune and Stratton, New York.

Hayhoe F.G.T. & Flemens R.J. (1982) *Haematological Cytology*, 2nd edition. Wolfe Medical, London.

Kay H.E.M. (1981) Acute Leukaemia. In *Recent Advances in Haematology 3*, ed. A.V. Hoffbrand. Churchill-Livingstone, Edinburgh.

Prentice H.G. (1983) A review of the current status and techniques of allogeneic bone marrow transplantation for treatment of leukaemia. *Journal of Clinical Pathology* **36,** 1207–14.

Rowley J.D. (1981) Cytogenetic studies in haematologic disorders. In *Recent Advances in Haematology 3*, ed. A.V. Hoffbrand. Churchill-Livingstone, Edinburgh.

Seminars in Hematology (1982) vol. 19, *Leukemia and Lymphoma*. Eds. R. Powles and T. McElwain. Grune and Stratton, New York.

Shaw M.T. (ed.) (1982) *Chronic Granulocytic Leukaemia*. Praeger Scientific, Eastbourne.

Warnke R.A. & Link M.P. (1983) Identification and significance of cell markers in leukaemia and lymphoma. *Annual Review of Medicine* **34,** 117–31.

Major textbooks of haematology (see Chapter 1).

Chapter 8
Malignant lymphomas

This group of diseases is divided into Hodgkin's disease and non-Hodgkin's lymphoma. In both, there is replacement of normal lymphoid structure by collections of abnormal cells, Hodgkin's disease being characterised by the presence of Reed–Sternberg (RS) cells and the non-Hodgkin's lymphomas by diffuse or nodular collection of abnormal lymphocytes or, rarely, histiocytes.

HODGKIN'S DISEASE

Pathogenesis

Hodgkin's disease is a malignant tumour closely related to the other malignant lymphomas. In many patients, the disease is localized initially to a single peripheral lymph node region and its subsequent progression is by contiguity within the lymphatic system. It is likely that the characteristic Reed–Sternberg cells and associated abnormal and smaller mononuclear cells (now thought to be derived from histiocytes) are neoplastic and that the associated inflammatory cells represent a hypersensitivity response by the host, the effectiveness of which determines the pattern of evolution. This aspect is further discussed under histological classification (see p. 155). After a variable period of containment within the lymph nodes, the natural progression of the disease is to disseminate to involve non-lymphatic tissue.

Clinical features

The disease can present at any age but it is rare in children and particularly frequent among young and middle-aged adults with an almost 2:1 male predominance.
(i) Most patients present with painless, non-tender asymmetrical, firm, discrete and rubbery enlargement of the superficial lymph nodes. The cervical nodes are involved in 60–70% of patients,

axillary nodes in about 10–15% and inguinal nodes in 6–12%. In some cases the size of the nodes decreases and increases spontaneously. They may become matted. Retroperitoneal nodes are also often involved but usually only diagnosed by laparotomy, lymphangiography or computerised axial tomography (CT scan).

(ii) Clinical splenomegaly occurs during the course of the disease in 50% of patients. The splenic enlargement is seldom massive. The liver may also be enlarged due to liver involvement.

(iii) Mediastinal involvement is found in 6–11% of patients at presentation. This is a feature of nodular sclerosis type, particularly in women. There may be associated pleural effusions or superior vena cava obstruction.

(iv) Cutaneous Hodgkin's disease occurs as a late complication in about 10% of patients. Other organs (e.g. gastrointestinal tract, bone, lung, spinal cord or brain) may also be involved even at presentation but this is unusual.

(v) Constitutional symptoms are prominent in patients with widespread disease. The following may be seen:

    a.   Fever occurs in about 30% of patients and is continuous or cyclic. In the latter type, a few days of high swinging pyrexia may alternate with a few days when the patient is afebrile (Pel–Ebstein fever) (Fig. 8.1).

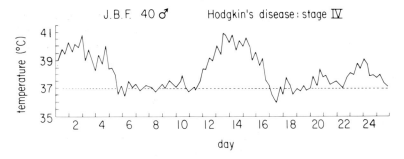

Fig. 8.1 A typical temperature chart in Hodgkin's disease (Pel–Ebstein fever).

    b.   Pruritus, which is often severe, occurs in about 25% of cases.

    c.   Alcohol-induced pain in the areas where disease is present occurs in some patients.

    d.   Other constitutional symptoms include weight loss, profuse sweating (especially at night), weakness, fatigue, anorexia and cachexia. Haematological and infectious complications are discussed below.

Haematological findings

(i) Normochromic, normocytic anaemia is most common. With marrow infiltration, bone marrow failure may occur with a leuco-erythroblastic anaemia.

(ii) One-third of patients have a leucocytosis due to a neutrophil increase.

(iii) The neutrophil alkaline phosphatase score is increased during the active phases of the disease.

(iv) Eosinophilia is frequent.

(v) Advanced disease is associated with lymphopenia.

(vi) The platelet count is normal or increased during early disease, and reduced in later stages.

(vii) The ESR is usually raised.

(viii) Bone marrow involvement is unusual in early disease but may be demonstrated by trephine biopsy, usually in patients with disease at many sites.

IMMUNOLOGICAL FINDINGS. There is a progressive loss of immunologically competent T-lymphocytes with reduced cell-mediated immune reactions. Antibody production is maintained until the later stages of the disease. Infections are common, particularly herpes zoster, cytomegalovirus and fungal, e.g. cryptococcus and candida. Tuberculosis may occur.

BIOCHEMICAL FINDINGS. Patients with bone disease may show hypercalcaemia, hypophosphataemia and increased levels of serum alkaline phosphatase. Elevated levels of serum transaminases may indicate liver involvement. Hyperuricaemia may occur.

Diagnosis and histological classification

The diagnosis is usually made by histological examination of an excised lymph node. The distinctive multinucleate polyploid Reed–Sternberg cell is central to the diagnosis (Fig. 8.2a & 8.2b). Inflammatory components consist of lymphocytes, histiocytes, polymorphs, eosinophils, plasma cells and variable fibrosis (Fig. 8.2b) Histological classification is into four types (Table 8.1), each of which implies a different prognosis. Patients with lymphocyte predominant histology have the most favourable prognosis. It is possible that they have a more effective cellular immune response than those with a lymphocyte depleted histology who have a relatively poor prognosis. Nodular sclerosis may be associated with each of the other three histological types and then carries the corresponding prognosis.

The nodular sclerosis type predominates in young adults, the other types have a bimodal age distribution with a second peak in old age. Lymphocyte predominance occurs mostly in children, lymphocyte depletion in the elderly.

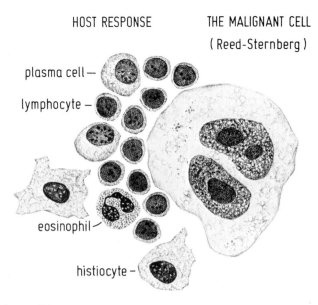

HOST RESPONSE   THE MALIGNANT CELL

(Reed-Sternberg)

plasma cell –

lymphocyte –

eosinophil –

histiocyte –

Fig. 8.2a Diagrammatic representation of the different cells seen histologically in Hodgkin's disease.

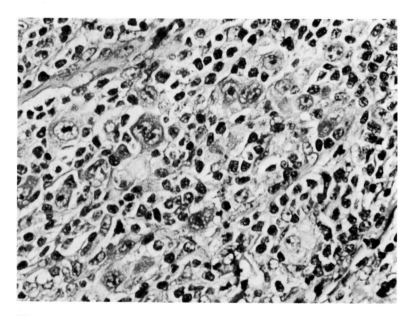

Fig. 8.2b Histological section of mixed cellularity Hodgkin's tissue.

Table 8.1 Histological classification of Hodgkin's disease.

Lymphocyte predominant
Lymphocyte proliferation dominates. Few Reed–Sternberg cells are seen. Nodular and diffuse patterns are recognised

Nodular sclerosis
Collagen bands extend from the node capsule to encircle nodules of abnormal tissue. A characteristic 'lacunar cell' variant of the Reed–Sternberg cell is often found. The cellular infiltrate may be of the lymphocyte predominant, mixed cellularity or lymphocyte depleted type.

Mixed cellularity
The Reed–Sternberg cells are numerous and lymphocyte numbers are intermediate (Fig. 8.2b)

Lymphocyte depleted
There is either a 'reticular' pattern with dominance of Reed–Sternberg cells and sparse numbers of lymphocytes or a 'diffuse fibrosis' pattern where the lymph node is replaced by disordered connective tissue containing few lymphocytes. Reed–Sternberg cells may also be infrequent in this latter sub-type

Clinical staging

Prognosis and selection of appropriate treatment depends on accurate staging of the extent of disease. Fig. 8.3 shows the scheme now recommended. Thorough clinical examination and the following procedures are employed:

Chest X-Ray to detect mediastinal, hilar node or lung involvement (Fig. 8.4a).

Bone marrow trephine biopsy.

Liver biopsy (percutaneous needle or wedge at laparotomy).

Spleen and liver isotope or ultrasound scanning to detect deposits or diffuse enlargement. CT scanning is used in some centres.

Lymphangiography may detect clinically silent pelvic and retroperitoneal para-aortic node involvement (Fig. 8.4b).

Staging laparotomy and splenectomy are used because of the unreliability of clinical staging employing the above methods. Many clinicians, therefore, advocate the performance of laparotomy with abdominal node and liver biopsy and splenectomy in all cases considered to be Stage I or II after clinical examination and the above tests.

The patients are also classified as 'A' or 'B' according to whether or not constitutional features (e.g. fever or weight loss) are present (see Fig. 8.3).

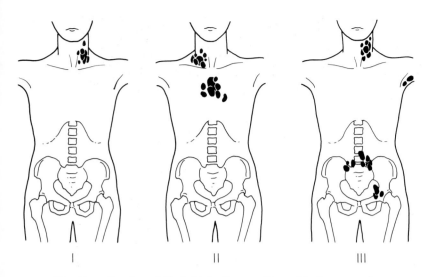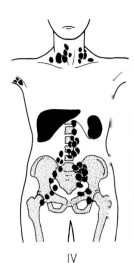

I II III IV

Fig. 8.3 Staging of Hodgkin's disease. *Stage I* indicates node involvement in one lymph node area. *Stage II* indicates disease involving two or more lymph nodal areas confined to one side of the diaphragm. *Stage III* indicates disease involving lymph nodes above and below the diaphragm. Splenic disease is included in stage *III* but this has special significance (see below). *Stage IV* indicates involvement outside the lymph node areas and refers to disease in the bone marrow, liver and other extranodal sites.

Note The stage number in all cases is followed by the letter A or B— indicating the absence (A) or presence (B) of one or more of the following: unexplained fever above 38°C; night sweats; and loss of more than 10% of body weight within six months. Localised extranodal extension from a mass of nodes does not advance the stage but is indicated by the subscript $_E$. Thus mediastinal disease with contiguous spread to the lung or spinal theca would be classified as I_E. As involvement of the spleen is often a prelude to widespread haematogenous spread of the disease, patients with lymph node and splenic involvement are staged as III_s.

Treatment

RADIOTHERAPY. This is the treatment of choice in patients with Stage I and II disease, and is also used in some Stage III and IV patients in combination with chemotherapy. Patients with Stage I and IIA Hodgkin's disease may be cured by radiotherapy alone. A total dose of not less than 4000 rads is able to destroy lymph node Hodgkin's tissue in most of these patients. Improved high voltage radiotherapy techniques allow the treatment of all lymph node areas above or below the diaphragm by single 'upper mantle' or 'inverted Y' blocks. Radiotherapy also has a role in treatment of particularly bulky tumour masses or painful skeletal, nodal or soft tissue deposits and ulcerating skin lesions in Stage II, III or IV patients following chemotherapy.

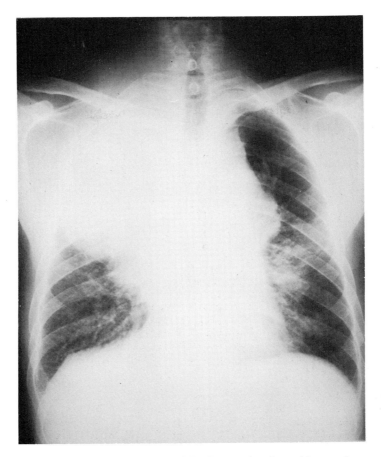

Fig. 8.4a Chest X-ray in Hodgkin's disease showing widespread enlargement of hilar and mediastinal lymph nodes with associated collapse of the right upper lobe and infiltration or possibly pneumonic changes in the mid zone of the left lung.

CHEMOTHERAPY. Cyclical chemotherapy is used for Stage III and IV disease and some also use it for patients with Stage IIB disease, or even Stage IIA if there is bulky disease involving three or more nodal sites. Quadruple therapy with Mustine, Vincristine (Oncovin), Procarbazine and Prednisolone (MOPP) has proved superior to single agent therapy. Other combinations have been used with equal success employing chlorambucil instead of mustine and vinblastine instead of vincristine. Other drugs, e.g. adriamycin and bleomycin, are usually reserved for resistant disease, e.g. in the combination ABVD (adriamycin, bleomycin, vinblastine, dacarbazine) although there is increasing use of them in initial therapy (e.g. alternating courses of MOPP and ABVD).

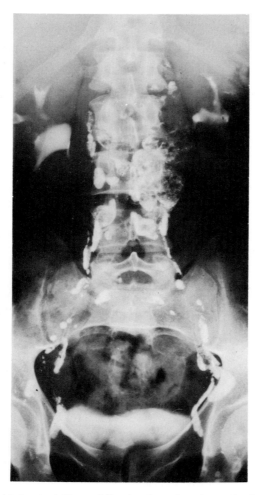

Fig. 8.4b Abdominal X-ray following lymphangiography in Hodgkin's
disease. There is marked enlargement of the para-aortic lymph nodes
with disruption of the normal nodal pattern. The pelvic lymph nodes
appear normal. An IVP, performed on the second day of the
lymphangiography study, demonstrates the relation of the kidneys and
ureters to the associated enlarged lymph nodes.

Prognosis

Approximate, 5 year survival rates are: Stages I and II: 85%; Stage
IIIA: 70%; Stages IIIB & IV: 50%.

As mentioned above, the histological grading also affects prognosis
within each of the clinical stages. There is a 5–10% incidence of
AML in patients surviving more than 5 years after treatment of
Hodgkin's disease with alkylating agents, especially if radiotherapy
has also been given.

NON-HODGKIN'S LYMPHOMA

The clinical presentation and natural history of these malignant lymphomas are more variable than in Hodgkin's disease, the pattern of spread is not as regular, and a greater proportion of patients present with extranodal disease or leukaemic manifestations.

Classification and histopathology

In recent years, no area of diagnostic histopathology has been associated with greater confusion than the classification of non-Hodgkin's lymphomas. The recognition that the majority of non-Hodgkin's lymphomas arise from germinal follicle centre cells (FCC) and that these tumours may have either follicular (nodular) or diffuse architecture, was a major conceptional advance in the understanding and classification. Lymphoid marker studies on tumour cells have also contributed to our knowledge. Although it is not without flaws, the Kiel classification based on the developmental cytology of the lymphoid system is used in this account. Table 8.2 gives this classification along with the older but popular classification of Rappaport.

A scheme of normal lymphocyte development appears in Fig. 6.8. In the Kiel classification, malignant lymphomas are named according to the supposed normal counterpart of the predominant tumour cell identified in histological sections and by imprint cytology. It is assumed that the tumour represents a clone of cells, whose maturation is fixed at a particular stage of development, with an inability to proceed further.

The non-Hodgkin's lymphomas are a diverse group of diseases varying from highly proliferative and rapidly fatal diseases, to some of the most indolent and well-tolerated malignancies in man. The Kiel classification recognises low-grade and high-grade malignancy groups. Patients with centrocytic and centroblastic lymphomas with a follicular pattern and patients with relatively small lymphoid cells (lymphocytes and lympho-plasmacytoid cells) have a more favourable natural history and survival. The high-grade malignancy group of tumours characterised by larger 'blast' forms carry with them a poor prognosis.

Practically all follicular and most diffuse lymphomas are derived from B-lymphocytes. Less than 10% carry membrane features of T-cells and a similar proportion have neither B- nor T-cell markers and are designated as 'null' cell tumours.

Lymphocytic lymphoma is closely related to chronic lymphocytic leukaemia and many regard this lymphoma as a tissue phase of this disease. The characteristic small, mature-appearing lymphocyte, rather than being 'well differentiated', is probably a so-called

Table 8.2 The classification of malignant lymphoma (FCC = follicle centre cell).

	Kiel (Lennert)		Rappaport
Low-grade malignancy	*Cell type*	*Variants*	*Nodular lymphomas*
	Lymphocytic	B + T cell (CLL), mycosis fungoides & Sézary syndrome	Lymphocytic, poorly differentiated
	Lymphoplasmacytoid/plasmacytic	B cell. Waldenström's macroglobulinaemia	Mixed lymphocytic histiocytic
			Histiocytic
	Centrocytic	FCC tumours of 'B' cell origin—follicular and diffuse patterns of involvement	*Diffuse lymphomas*
	Centrocytic/centroblastic		Lymphocytic, well differentiated
High-grade malignancy	Centroblastic		Lymphocytic, poorly differentiated
	Immunoblastic	B + T cell subtypes 'null', B + T cell variants, Burkitt's lymphoma	Mixed lymphocytic histiocytic
	Lymphoblastic		Histiocytic
			Undifferentiated
			Burkitt-type
			Non-Burkitt-type
Monocytic-macrophage system tumours	True 'histiocytic' lymphoma	Histiocytic medullary reticulosis	
	Malignant histiocytosis		

'virgin' B-cell which has not been stimulated by antigen to react and divide. Many patients with this condition are elderly with slowly progressive disease, which may not require treatment for extended periods. Some lympho-plasmacytoid lymphomas may be associated with the production of monoclonal paraproteins. If there are significant amounts of IgM, the condition is known as Waldenström's macroglobulinaemia (see p. 178).

Patients with follicular tumours are likely to be middle-aged and their disease is often characterised by a benign course for many years. However, sudden transformation may occur to aggressive blast cell and diffuse tumours which are sometimes associated with a leukaemic phase.

The blastic or high-grade malignancy group of lymphomas are associated with a fast rate of cellular proliferation. Histologically, in immunoblastic and centroblastic types, there is widespread destruction of nodal architecture often with extension through the capsule to surrounding perinodal tissues. Progressive infiltration may affect the gastrointestinal tract, the spinal cord, the kidneys or other organs. The lymphoblastic lymphomas occur mainly in children and young adults and these conditions merge clinically and morphologically with acute lymphoblastic leukaemia of the poor prognosis type. Young patients presenting with mediastinal masses may be labelled as T-cell lymphoblastic lymphoma or Thy-cell lymphoblastic leukaemia (Thy-ALL) depending on the degree of bone marrow and peripheral blood involvement at presentation.

It is now clear from marker studies, that tumours of true 'histiocytes' or monocyte-derived cells are rare. These tumours carry a poor prognosis and require intensive chemotherapy but with this some patients may be cured. In histiocytic medullary reticulosis, the malignant cells are true histiocytes which proliferate rapidly and phagocytose red cells causing a haemolytic anaemia.

Clinical features

The median age at presentation is 50.

(i) *Superficial lymphadenopathy.* The majority of patients present with asymmetric painless enlargement of lymph nodes in one or more peripheral lymph node region.

(ii) *Constitutional symptoms.* Fever, night sweats and weight loss occur less frequently than in Hodgkin's disease and their presence is usually associated with disseminated disease. Anaemia and infections of the type seen in Hodgkin's disease may occur.

(iii) *Oropharyngeal involvement.* In 5–10% of patients there is disease of oropharyngeal lymphoid structures (Waldeyer's ring) which may cause complaints of a 'sore throat' or noisy or obstructed breathing.

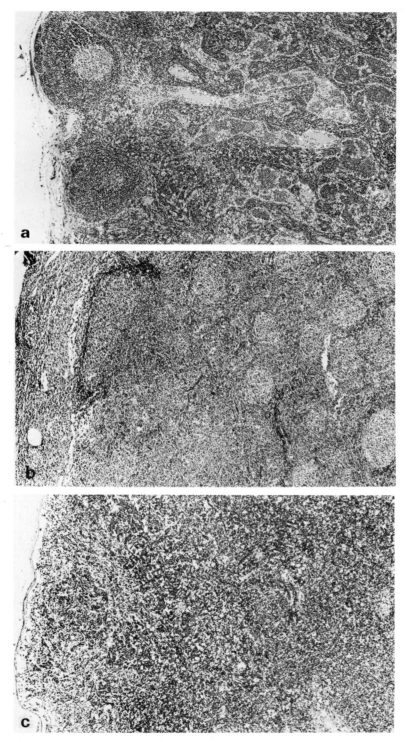

Fig. 8.5 Low power magnification sections of: **a** normal lymph node, **b** 'follicular' pattern non-Hodgkin's lymphoma, and **c** 'diffuse' pattern non-Hodgkin's lymphoma. All stained with haematoxylin and eosin.

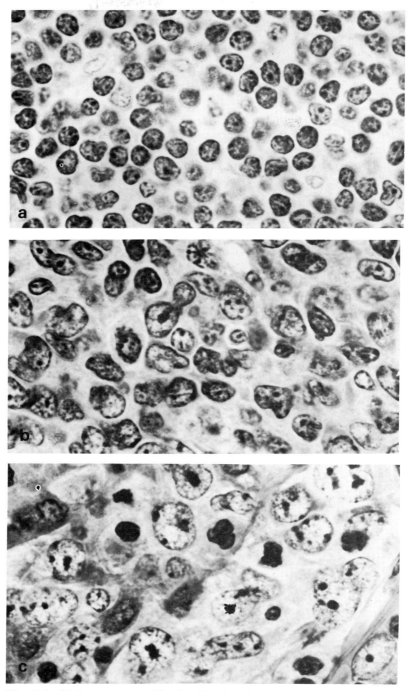

Fig. 8.6 High power magnification histology in non-Hodgkin's
lymphoma stained with haematoxylin and eosin,
a Lymphocytic lymphoma. The majority of cells are small lymphocytes;
b Centroblastic/centrocytic lymphoma. The cells are similar to their
counterparts seen in a normal follicular germinal centre;
c Immunoblastic lymphoma. The cells are large pleomorphic
immunoblasts with prominent nuclei.

(iv) *Anaemia*, infections or purpura may be presenting features in patients with diffuse bone marrow disease.

(v) *Abdominal disease*. The liver and spleen are often enlarged and involvement of retroperitoneal or mesenteric nodes is frequent (Fig. 8.8). The gastrointestinal tract is the most commonly involved extranodal site after the bone marrow and patients may present with acute abdominal symptoms.

(vi) *Other organs*. Skin, brain, testis or thyroid involvement is not infrequent. The skin is also primarily involved in two unusual closely related T cell lymphomas, mycosis fungoides and Sézary's syndrome.

Haematological findings

(i) A normochromic, normocytic anaemia is usual but auto-immune haemolytic anaemia may also occur.

(ii) In advanced disease with marrow involvement there may be neutropenia, thrombocytopenia or leuco-erythroblastic features.

(iii) Lymphoma cells ('follicular lymphoma' or 'lymphosarcoma'

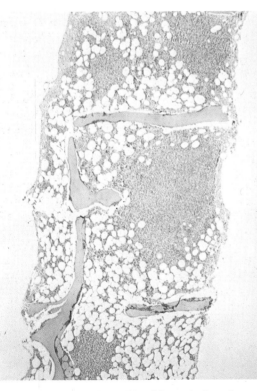

Fig. 8.7 Iliac crest trephine biopsy in lymphocytic lymphoma. Four prominent nodules of lymphoid tissue are seen in the intertrabecular space.

cells) with variable nuclear abnormalities may be found in the peripheral blood in some patients.

(iv) Trephine biopsy of marrow shows focal involvement in about 20% of cases (Fig. 8.7). Diffuse infiltration accompanied by fibrosis may also occur. Paradoxically, bone marrow involvement will be found more frequently in the low-grade malignancy lymphomas. Immunological marker studies using fluorescence or peroxidase techniques may detect minimal involvement not easily recognised by conventional microscopy.

IMMUNOLOGICAL FINDINGS. Lymphocyte marker studies show that the majority of malignant lymphomas are monoclonal B-cell tumours and occasionally there is an associated monoclonal paraprotein — usually IgM or IgG. In a few patients, particularly children with a mediastinal mass and lymphoblastic morphology, the disease is thymic in origin, and other tumours, e.g. Sézary's syndrome, consist of more mature T-cells. A few tumours can be shown to be truly histiocytic based on morphological, cytochemical and immunological criteria.

BLOOD CHEMISTRY. Elevation of serum uric acid may occur. Abnormal liver function tests suggest disseminated disease.

Diagnostic investigations and clinical staging

The diagnosis is made by histological examination of excised lymph nodes (see Fig. 8.5) or extranodal tumour and attempts are made accurately to stage the extent of the disease. The staging system is the same as that described for Hodgkin's disease but is less clearly related than histological type to prognosis.

Other staging procedures include chest X-rays to detect thoracic involvement, liver biopsy, lymphangiography, isotopic, ultrasonic or CT scanning (Fig. 8.8) to detect abdominal disease and bone marrow aspiration and trephine (Fig. 8.7).

Exploratory laparotomy and splenectomy. Because of the early haematogenous spread in the majority of patients with non-Hodgkin's lymphoma there is usually no need for these procedures in non-Hodgkin's lymphomas, except when required to make the initial diagnosis.

Localised extranodal disease and staging. In 10–15% of patients there is initial extranodal disease, e.g. involvement of the gastrointestinal tract, lung and other organs such as the skin, brain or testis. If a careful search fails to show evidence of disseminated disease these patients are graded as having Stage I_E rather than Stage IV.

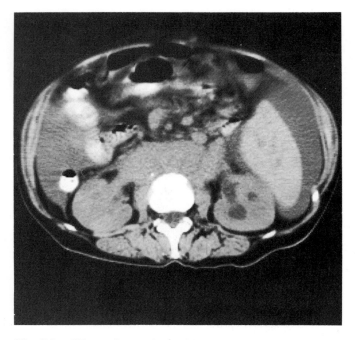

Fig. 8.8 CT scan in a patient with non-Hodgkin's lymphoma showing massive enlargement of retroperitoneal lymph nodes.

Treatment

The approach to treatment varies with the type of disease. Some patients with low-grade malignancy tumours, particularly the lymphocytic group, require no initial treatment if they are asymptomatic and the size or location of the lymphadenopathy poses no major threat.

RADIOTHERAPY

Although some patients with truly localised Stage I disease may be cured by radiotherapy, there is a high rate of early relapse in patients classified as Stage II or III disease. Local radiation for major bulky sites of the disease should be considered in patients receiving chemotherapy and this may be especially useful if the disease is resulting in anatomical obstruction.

In patients with Stage III and IV low-grade malignancy lymphomas, palliative low dose total body irradiation may produce results comparable to those of chemotherapy.

1 *Single agent therapy.* Continuous or intermittent chlorambucil or cyclophosphamide may produce good results in patients with lymphomas of low-grade malignancy who require therapy because of advancing disease or systemic symptoms.

2 *Combination therapy* (e.g. cyclophosphamide, vincristine and prednisolone (COP)) may also be used in patients with low- or intermediate-grade disease based on histological and clinical staging.

Intensive cyclical chemotherapy improves survival rates in patients who have high-grade malignancy lymphomas of clinical Stages II, III and IV. Paradoxically, prolonged disease-free survival and cure is possible, despite their poor natural history. Daunorubicin or hydroxodaunorubicin and/or bleomycin are added to the cyclophosphamide, vincristine and prednisone in some of the regimens (CHOP or B-CHOP) and even more intensive regimens are being used—adding high dose methotrexate.

Patients with lymphoblastic lymphoma are treated with intensive chemotherapy programmes similar to those used for poor prognosis childhood acute lymphoblastic leukaemia. Central nervous system prophylaxis employing intrathecal (or high dose systemic) methotrexate and cranial irradiation is required to prevent meningeal relapse in young subjects.

Prognosis

The majority of patients with low-grade malignant disease and follicular patterns of architecture survive for longer than five years and many are alive more than ten years from the time of diagnosis. Many patients with localised high-grade malignancy disease are cured by radiotherapy. With intensive chemotherapy, patients with widespread high-grade malignant lymphomas have a 40–50% disease-free survival at two years and it seems likely that some of these patients will have prolonged survival and may be cured.

BURKITT ('AFRICAN') LYMPHOMA

This unusual (B-lymphoblastic) lymphoma which is found particularly in young African children has a peculiar predilection for massive jaw lesions, extranodal abdominal involvement and, in girls, ovarian tumours.

Isolated histiocytes in the masses of abnormal lymphoblasts produce a characteristic 'starry sky' appearance in tissue sections. The Epstein–Barr virus has been identified in Burkitt cell culture and the chromosome translocation $14q^+ 8q^-$ is usual.

Chemotherapy produces dramatic initial clinical remissions but relapses are frequent, with only 30% of patients being cured.

ANGIOIMMUNOBLASTIC LYMPHADENOPATHY

This disease usually occurs in elderly patients with generalised lymphadenopathy, hepatosplenomegaly, skin rashes and a polyclonal increase in serum IgG. Occasionally, the condition appears to be precipitated by exposure to drugs. Histologically, the lymph node shows replacement by a mixed cellular infiltrate, comprising immunoblasts, plasma cells, macrophages and granulocytes, around proliferating small blood vessels. The condition may transform into an immunoblastic lymphoma.

Table 8.3 Causes of lymphadenopathy.

Localised
Local infection
    pyogenic infection (e.g. pharyngitis, dental abscess, otitis media)
    viral infection (e.g. cat scratch fever, lymphogranuloma venereum)
    tuberculosis
    fungal infections (e.g. actinomycosis)
Lymphoma
    Hodgkin's disease
    Non-Hodgkin's lymphoma
Carcinoma (secondary)

Generalised
Infections
    viral (e.g. infectious mononucleosis, measles, rubella, viral hepatitis)
    bacterial (e.g. brucellosis, syphilis, tuberculosis, salmonella, bacterial endocarditis)
    fungal (e.g. histoplasmosis)
    protozoal (e.g. toxoplasmosis)

Non-infectious inflammatory diseases (e.g. sarcoidosis, rheumatoid arthritis, systemic lupus erythematosus, other connective tissue diseases, serum sickness)
Leukaemias, especially CLL, ALL
Lymphoma: non-Hodgkin's lymphoma, Hodgkin's disease
Rarely secondary carcinoma
Angioimmunoblastic lymphadenopathy
Sinus histocytosis with massive lymphadenopathy
Reaction to drugs and chemicals (e.g. hydantoins and related chemicals, beryllium)
Hyperthyroidism

SINUS HISTIOCYTOSIS WITH MASSIVE LYMPHADENOPATHY

This occurs particularly in young Negroes and is characterised by massive cervical lymphadenopathy, fever, leucocytosis and a polyclonal increase in IgG. The nodes show sinusoidal dilation with plasma cell and macrophage infiltration. The condition appears to be due to virus infection and recovers spontaneously usually over several months or years.

MYCOSIS FUNGOIDES AND SEZARY'S SYNDROME

Mycosis fungoides is a chronic cutaneous T-cell lymphoma which presents with severe pruritus and psoriaform lesions. Ultimately deeper organs are affected, particularly lymph nodes, spleen, liver and bone marrow. In Sézary's syndrome, there is characteristically exfoliative dermatitis, erythrodermia, generalised lymphadenopathy and circulating T-lymphoma cells. Initial treatment of these conditions is by local irradiation, topical chemotherapy or PUVA.

ADULT T-CELL LEUKAEMIA/LYMPHOMA

This is a widespread disease of adults of either sex, usually presenting with lymphadenopathy, hepatic and splenic enlargement, cutaneous infiltrations and hypercalcaemia. The disease is frequent in Japan, the Caribbean and South America but occurs in countries of Africa, the USA and sporadically elsewhere. It has a rapid clinical course. The blood, bone marrow and other tissues are infiltrated with lymphoma cells with lobulated nuclei, which have been shown to be T-cells infected with human T-cell leukaemia/lymphoma virus, HTLV-I.

The virus is an exogenous human chronic leukaemia retrovirus. The site of integration into the host cell DNA varies between patients, but in any one patient, is clonal. Serological studies show that many apparently healthy persons have also been infected with the virus and are carriers. They are found most frequently among close contacts of the patients with overt disease. The mechanism by which the virus causes malignant transformation in a proportion of infected subjects is uncertain since the virus lacks a transforming oncogene (v-onc).

Close contact appears to be necesary for HTLV-I transmission. A related virus, HTLV-III is now thought to be the cause of

AIDS. The AIDS virus also infects T-cells, specifically of the T_4 subset, but kills them, leading to immune suppression rather than to malignant transformation.

DIFFERENTIAL DIAGNOSIS OF LYMPHADENOPATHY

The principal causes of lymphadenopathy are listed in Table 8.3. The clinical history and examination give essential information. The age of the patient, the length of history, associated symptoms of possible infection or malignant disease, whether the nodes are painful of tender, the consistency of the nodes and whether there is generalised or local lymphadenopathy, are all important. The size of the liver and spleen are assessed. In the case of local node enlargement, inflammatory or malignant disease in the associated lymphatic drainage area is particularly considered.

Further investigations will depend on the initial clinical diagnosis but it is usual to include a full blood count, blood film and ESR. Chest X-ray, Paul–Bunnell, toxoplasma titres and Mantoux testing are frequently needed. In many cases, it will be essential to make a histological diagnosis by node biopsy but a fine needle aspirate may sometimes avoid the need for this. Subsequent investigations will depend on the diagnosis made and the patient's particular features. In some cases of deep node enlargement, where enlarged superficial nodes are not available for biopsy, bone marrow or liver biopsies may be needed in an attempt to reach a histological diagnosis and avoid the need for a diagnostic laparotomy.

SELECTED BIBLIOGRAPHY

Clinics in Haematology (1979) vol. 8.3, *The Non-Hodgkin's Lymphomas*. Ed. G.P. Canellos. W.B. Saunders, Philadelphia.

Kaplan H.S. (1980) *Hodgkin's Disease*, 2nd edition. Harvard University Press, Cambridge, Mass.

Lennert K. (1981) *Malignant Lymphomas other than Hodgkin's Disease*. Springer Verlag, New York.

Rappaport H. (1977) Histological classification: non-Hodgkin's lymphoma. In *Cancer Treatment Reports*, eds. S.E. Janes & T. Grodden. **61**, 1037–48.

Robb-Smith A.H.T. & Taylor C.R. (1981) *Lymph Node Biopsy*. Miller Heyden, London.

Stein H. *et al* (1982) The normal and malignant germinal centre. *Clinics in Haematology*, vol. 11.3, pp. 531–60. W.B. Saunders, Philadelphia.

Wright D.H. (1982) The identification and classification of non-Hodgkin's lymphoma: a review. *Diagnostic Histopathology* **5**, 73–111.

Major textbooks of haematology (see Chapter 1).

Chapter 9
Multiple myeloma

Multiple myeloma (myelomatosis) is a neoplastic monoclonal proliferation of bone marrow plasma cells, characterised by lytic bone
lesions, plasma cell accumulation in the bone marrow, and the
presence of monoclonal protein in serum and urine. Eighty per cent
of cases occur over the age of 40. In Britain there is a mean annual
death rate of 9 per million of the population.

Clinical features

(i) Bone pain (especially backache), pathological fractures.
(ii) Of anaemia: lethargy, weakness, dyspnoea, pallor, tachycardia, etc.
(iii) Repeated infections: these are related to deficient antibody
production and, in advanced disease, to neutropenia.
(iv) Of renal failure and/or hypercalcaemia: polydipsia, polyuria,
anorexia, vomiting, constipation and mental disturbance.
(v) Abnormal bleeding tendency: myeloma protein interferes
with platelet function and coagulation factors; thrombocytopenia
occurs in advanced disease.
(vi) Occasionally there is macroglossia, 'carpal tunnel syndrome'
and diarrhoea due to amyloid disease.
(vii) Rarely there is a 'hyperviscosity syndrome' with purpura,
haemorrhages, visual failure, CNS symptoms and neuropathies,
and heart failure. This results from polymerisation of the
abnormal immunoglobulin and is particularly likely when this is
IgA, IgM, or IgD.

Diagnosis

This depends on three principal findings. In 98% of patients monoclonal protein occurs in the serum or urine or both (Fig. 9.1). The
serum paraprotein is IgG in two-thirds, IgA in one-third, with rare
IgM or IgD or mixed cases. Other causes of a serum paraprotein
are listed in Table 9.1. In doubtful cases, follow-up studies will
show a progressive rise in paraprotein concentrations in untreated

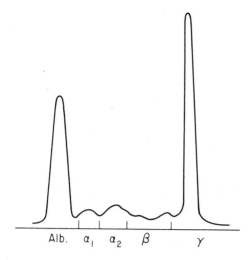

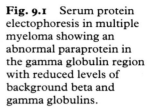

Fig. 9.1 Serum protein electophoresis in multiple myeloma showing an abnormal paraprotein in the gamma globulin region with reduced levels of background beta and gamma globulins.

Alb. α_1 α_2 β γ

myeloma. Normal serum immunoglobulins (IgG, IgA, and IgM) are depressed. The urine contains Bence-Jones protein in two-thirds of cases. This consists of free light chains, either kappa or lambda, of the same type as the serum paraprotein. In 15% of cases, however, Bence-Jones proteinuria is present without a serum paraprotein.

The bone marrow shows increased plasma cells ($>10\%$ and usually more than 30%), often with abnormal forms—'myeloma cells' (Fig. 9.2). Immunological testing shows these cells to be monoclonal and to express the same immunoglobulin chains as the serum monoclonal protein.

Skeletal survey shows osteolytic areas without evidence of surrounding osteoblastic reaction or sclerosis in 60% of patients (Fig. 9.3) or generalised bone rarefaction (20%). Pathological fractures are common. No lesions are found in 20% of patients. Usually at least two of the three diagnostic features mentioned above are present.

OTHER LABORATORY FINDINGS

(i) There is usually a normochromic normocytic or macrocytic anaemia. Rouleaux formation is marked in most cases (Fig. 9.4). Neutropenia and thrombocytopenia occur in advanced disease.

Table 9.1 Causes of a paraprotein.

Benign monoclonal gammopathy
Multiple myeloma
Macroglobulinaemia
Malignant lymphoma or chronic lymphocytic leukaemia
Chronic cold haemagglutinin disease (see p. 82)
Rarely with carcinoma

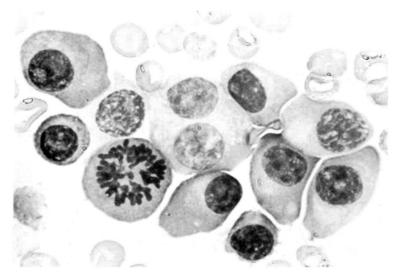

Fig. 9.2 The bone marrow in multiple myeloma showing large numbers of plasma cells, with many abnormal forms.

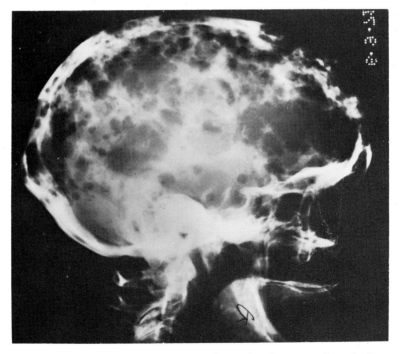

Fig. 9.3 Skull X-ray in multiple myeloma showing many 'punched-out' lesions.

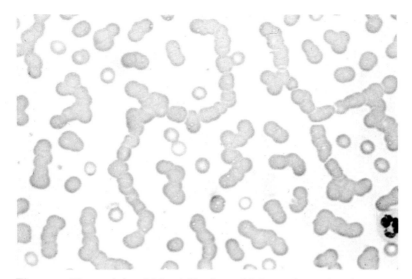

Fig. 9.4 The peripheral blood film in multiple myeloma showing rouleaux formation.

Abnormal plasma cells appear in blood film in 15% of patients. Leuco-erythroblastic changes are occasionally seen.
(ii) High ESR.
(iii) Serum calcium elevation occurs in 45% of patients. There is a normal serum alkaline phosphatase (except following pathological fractures).
(iv) The blood urea is raised above 14 mmol/l and serum creatinine raised in 20% of cases. Proteinaceous deposits from heavy Bence-Jones proteinuria, hypercalcaemia, uric acid, amyloid and pyelonephritis may all contribute to renal failure (Fig. 9.5).
(v) A low serum albumin occurs with advanced disease.

Treatment

EMERGENCY SITUATIONS
(i) Uraemia: rehydrate, treat underlying cause (e.g. hypercalcaemia, hyperuricaemia). Haemodialysis is considered in some patients.
(ii) Acute hypercalcaemia: hydration, prednisolone, phosphates

Fig. 9.5 (*opposite*) The kidney in multiple myeloma: **a** '*Myeloma kidney*'—the renal tubules are distended with hyaline protein (precipitated light chains or Bence-Jones protein). Giant cells are prominent in the surrounding cellular reaction. **b** *Amyloid deposition*—both glomeruli and several of the small blood vessels contain an amorphous dark-staining deposit characteristic of amyloid (Congo red stain). **c** '*Nephrocalcinosis*'—calcium deposition (dark 'fractured' material) in the renal parenchyma.

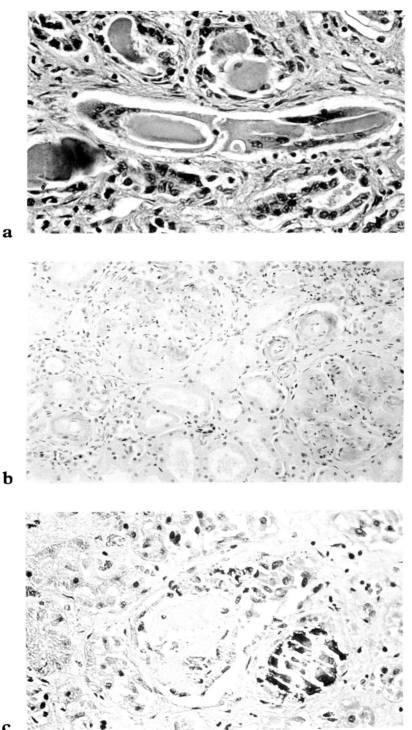

a

b

c

(intravenously or orally). Mithramycin or calcitonin may also be beneficial.

(iii) Compression paraplegia: decompression laminectomy, irradiation, chemotherapy.

(iv) Single painful skeletal lesion: chemotherapy or irradiation.

(v) Severe anaemia: transfusion of packed red cells.

(vi) Bleeding due to paraprotein interference with coagulation, and hyperviscosity syndrome may be treated by repeated plasmapheresis.

CHEMOTHERAPY. Alkylating agents relieve pain, reduce plasma cell proliferation in the marrow and so reduce the serum paraprotein levels. As plasma cells are killed, normal bone marrow function improves. Melphalan or cyclophosphamide, with or without prednisolone, are the drugs of choice. Melphalan is given daily for 4–7 days every 6–8 weeks. Allopurinol is also given to prevent urate nephropathy. Because of the inevitability of resistance developing to alkylating agent therapy, treatment of symptomless patients with early disease is not justified. Regular clinical and laboratory assessment should be made of disease progression. Treatment may be delayed until the development of signs or symptoms of bone marrow failure, until there is a rise in blood urea or Bence-Jones protein appears in the urine, or until bone lesions are extensive or cause symptoms.

Patients eventually become resistant to treatment; other drugs are then often tried, e.g. vincristine, adriamycin, bleomycin and nitrosoureas.

Prognosis

The median survival is two years with a 20% four year survival. The most serious prognostic feature is the blood urea concentration: if the blood urea is more than 14 mmol/l at presentation the median survival is only a few months. If the blood urea is less than 7 mmol/l at presentation the median survival is 33 months. Severe anaemia, a low serum albumin at presentation, and heavy Bence-Jones proteinuria are also bad prognostic features.

WALDENSTRÖM'S MACROGLOBULINAEMIA

This is an uncommon condition, seen most frequently in men over 50 years of age, which behaves clinically as a slowly progressive lymphoma. There is proliferation of cells which produce a monoclonal IgM paraprotein and bear some resemblance both to lymphocytes and plasma cells.

The term Waldenström's macroglobulinaemia is often restricted to cases where the dominant clinical features are the result of macroglobulinaemia and diffuse cellular infiltrates. Those cases with dominant tumour masses are often referred to as 'malignant lymphoma with macroglobulinaemia'. In both cases, the malignant cells is a monoclonal B-cell population.

Clinical features

(i) There is usually an insidious onset, with fatigue and weight loss.

(ii) Hyperviscosity syndrome may result in visual disturbances, lethargy, confusion, muscle weakness, nervous system symptoms and signs, and congestive heart failure. IgM paraprotein increases blood viscosity more than equivalent concentrations of IgG or IgA and small increases above 30 g/l in concentration lead to large increases in viscosity. The retina may show a variety of changes; engorged veins, haemorrhages, exudates and a blurred disc.

If the macroglubulin is a cryoglobulin, features of cryoprecipitations, e.g. Raynaud's phenomenon, may be present.

(iii) A bleeding tendency may result from macroglobulin interference with coagulation factors and platelet function.

(iv) Anaemia due to haemodilution, decreased red cell survival, blood loss and bone marrow failure in advanced disease.

(v) Moderate lymphadenopathy and enlargement of the liver and spleen are frequently seen.

Diagnosis

(i) Serum monoclonal IgM is usually greater than 15 g/l.

(ii) Bone marrow shows pleomorphic infiltration by small lymphocytes, plasma cells, 'plasmacytoid' forms, immature lymphoid cells, mast cells and histiocytes. Trephine biopsy may show more nodular disease which implies a better prognosis than the diffuse infiltration.

(iii) High ESR.

(iv) Often a peripheral blood lymphocytosis with some plasmacytoid lymphocytes.

(v) Lymph node histology shows sinus architecture preserved, loss of follicular pattern with cellular infiltration similar to that found in the bone marrow.

Treatment

(i) Acute hyperviscosity syndrome: repeated plasmapheresis. As IgM is mainly intravascular, this is more effective than with IgG or IgA paraproteins when much of the protein is extravascular and so rapidly replenishes the plasma compartment.

(ii) Supportive therapy; transfusions for anaemia, antibiotics for infections, etc.

(iii) The alkylating agent cyclophosphamide with prednisolone is the most widely used drug; it reduces bone marrow infiltration and lowers the serum concentration of IgM.

HEAVY-CHAIN DISEASES

These are rare syndromes characterised by the production of the α, γ or μ heavy chain of immunoglobulin and soft tissue tumours appearing histologically either as malignant lymphoma or plasmacytoma. α chain disease usually shows the clinical features of malabsorption due to intestinal infiltration.

BENIGN MONOCLONAL GAMMOPATHY

A paraprotein may be found in the serum, particularly of older subjects with no definite evidence of myeloma, macroglobulinaemia or lymphoma. There are no bone lesions, usually no Bence-Jones proteinuria, and the proportion of plasma cells in the marrow is normal (less than 4%) or only slightly raised (less than 10%). The concentration of monoclonal immunoglobulin in serum is usually less than 20 g/l and remains stationary when followed over a period of 2 or 3 years. Other serum immunoglobulins are not depressed. After many years of follow-up, however, a substantial proportion of these patients develop overt myeloma.

AMYLOIDOSIS

This is a homogenous deposit in tissues, staining pink with haematoxylin and eosin and red with Congo red, and exhibiting green birefringence. Amyloid has a fibrillary structure and is classified as follows.

Amyloid associated with monoclonal immunocyte proliferation

This type consists of light chains and/or the N terminal V_L domain of the light chain. This is termed the 'AL' type and occurs in association with myeloma, Waldenström's macroglobulinaemia, heavy-chain disease and in a 'primary' form. The clinical features are due to involvement of the heart, tongue, peripheral nerves and kidneys, and the patient may present with heart failure, macroglossia, peripheral neuropathy or the carpal tunnel syndrome, or with renal failure.

Reactive systemic amyloidosis

This type consists of a protein 'A' which is probably derived from an acute phase protein and is termed the 'AA' type. It occurs in association with chronic infections (e.g. tuberculosis), rheumatoid arthritis and neoplastic diseases, including Hodgkin's disease. It is also common in association with familial Mediterranean fever. The clinical features are due to reticulo-endothelial involvement with enlargement of the liver and spleen; kidney involvement may occur with renal vein thrombosis and the nephrotic syndrome.

Localised amyloid

This may occur around tumours, particularly of the endocrine system and also occurs in the skin and elsewhere in old age.

HYPERVISCOSITY SYNDROME

The commonest cause is polycythaemia (see p. 184). As already mentioned, hyperviscosity may also be a problem in patients with either myeloma or Waldenström's macroglobulinaemia. Occasionally it may also occur in patients with chronic granulocytic or acute leukaemia associated with very high white cell counts. Rarely, haemophilic patients with circulating inhibitors, being treated with massive doses of cryoprecipitate have developed hyperviscosity because of the large volumes of fibrinogen infused.

The clinical features of hyperviscosity syndrome have been described on p. 179. Emergency treatment varies with the cause: venesection or isovolaemic exchange of a plasma substitute for red cells in a polycythaemic patient; plasmapheresis in myeloma, Waldenström's disease or hyperfibrinogenaemia; leucopheresis in leukaemias associated with high white counts. The long-term treatment depends on control of the primary disease with specific therapy.

SELECTED BIBLIOGRAPHY

Clinics in Haematology (1977) Vol. 6.2, *Disorders of Lymphopoiesis and Lymphoid Function*. Ed. H.H. Fundenberg. W.B. Saunders, Philadelphia.

Clinics in Haematology (1982) vol. 11.1, *Myeloma and Related Disorders*. Ed. S.E. Salman. W.B. Saunders, Philadelphia.

Galton D.A.G. (1981) Myelomatosis. In *Postgraduate Haematology*, eds. A.V. Hoffbrand & S.M. Lewis. Heinemann, London.

Seminars in Hematology (1982) vol. 19, *Leukemia and Lymphoma*. Eds. R. Powles & T. McElwain. Grune and Stratton, New York.

Major textbooks of haematology (see Chapter 1).

Chapter 10
Myeloproliferative disorders

The term 'myeloproliferative disorders' describes a group of conditions characterised by endogenous proliferation of one or more haemopoietic component in the bone marrow and, in many cases, the liver and spleen. These disorders are closely related, transitional forms occur and, in many patients, an evolution from one entity into another occurs during the course of the disease (Fig. 10.1a). Polycythaemia vera, essential thrombocythaemia and myelosclerosis are collectively known as the 'non-leukaemic myeloproliferative disorders' and are discussed here; the myeloid leukaemias are discussed in Chapter 7.

POLYCYTHAEMIA VERA

Polycythaemia (erythrocytosis) refers to a pattern of blood cell changes that usually includes an increase in haemoglobin above 17.5 g/dl in males and 15.5 g/dl in females with an accompanying rise in red cell count (above $6.0 \times 10^{12}/l$ in males; $5.5 \times 10^{12}/l$ in females) and haematocrit (above 55% in males; 47% in females). The causes of polycythaemia are listed in Table 10.1 Studies with ^{51}Cr- or ^{99m}Tc-labelled red cells to measure total red cell volume (TRCV) and ^{125}I-albumin (to measure plasma volume) are required to establish whether the polycythaemia is 'real', where there is an increase in TRCV, or 'relative', where there is no increase in TRCV but the circulating plasma volume is decreased (Table 10.1). Polycythaemia is considered 'real' if the TRCV is greater than 36 ml kg^{-1} in men and 32 ml kg^{-1} in women (Table 10.2).

In polycythaemia vera (polycythaemia rubra vera, PV), the increase in red cell volume is caused by endogenous myeloproliferation. The stem cell nature of the defect is suggested in many patients by an overproduction of granulocytes and platelets as well as of red cells.

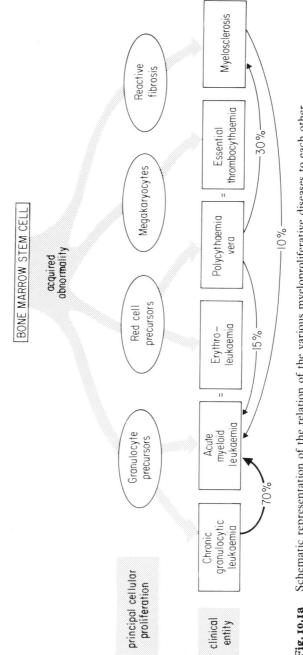

Fig. 10.1a Schematic representation of the relation of the various myeloproliferative diseases to each other. Many transitional cases occur showing features of two conditions and, in other cases, the disease transforms during its course from one of these diseases to another. Chronic granulocytic leukaemia may also transform into ALL.

Table 10.1 Causes of polycythaemia.

Primary
Polycythaemia vera *: Benign familial erythrocytosis .*

Secondary
Due to <u>compensatory erythropoietin increase</u> in:
  High altitudes
  Cardiovascular disease, especially congenital with cyanosis
  Pulmonary disease and alveolar hypoventilation
  Increased affinity haemoglobins (familial polycythaemia) (see Chapter
    4)
  Heavy smoking
  Methaemoglobinaemia (rarely)
Due to <u>inappropriate erythropoietin increase</u> in:
  Renal diseases, e.g. hydronephrosis, vascular impairment, cysts,
    carcinoma
  Massive uterine fibromyomata
  Hepatocellular carcinoma
  Cerebellar haemangioblastoma.

Relative
  'Stress' or 'spurious' polycythaemia
  Dehydration: water deprivation, vomiting
  Plasma loss: burns, enteropathy

(margin note: Hypoxia)

Table 10.2 Normal blood volume: radiodilution methods.

Total red cell volume (^{51}Cr or ^{99m}Tc)	Men	25–35 ml/kg
	Women	22–32 ml/kg
Total plasma volume (^{125}I-albumin):		40–50 ml/kg

(margin note: NB; Red PRV. >36ml/kg >32ml/kg)

Clinical features

This is a <u>disease of older subjects</u> with an <u>equal sex incidence</u>.
Clinical features are the result of <u>hyperviscosity</u>, <u>hypervolaemia</u>
or <u>hypermetabolism</u>.
(i) Headaches, <u>pruritus</u> (especially after a hot bath), dyspnoea,
blurred vision and night sweats.
(ii) Plethoric appearance—ruddy cyanosis, conjuctival suf-
fusion, retinal venous engorgement.
(iii) Splenomegaly in two-thirds of patients.
(iv) Haemorrhage (e.g. gastrointestinal, uterine, cerebral) or
thrombosis either arterial (e.g. cardiac, cerebral, peripheral) or
venous (e.g. deep or superficial leg veins, cerebral, portal or
hepatic veins) are frequent.
(v) Hypertension in one-third of patients.
(vi) Gout (due to raised uric acid production (Fig. 10.1b)).
(vii) Peptic ulceration occurs in 5–10% of patients.

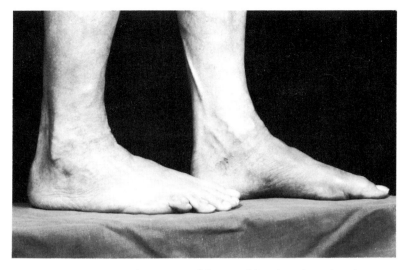

Fig. 10.1b The feet of a 72-year-old man with polycythaemia rubra vera. There is inflammation of the left metatarso-phalangeal and other joints due to uric acid deposits.

Laboratory features

(i) The haemoglobin, haematocrit and red cell count are increased. The total red cell volume is increased.

(ii) A neutrophil leucocytosis is seen in over half the patients, and some have increased circulating basophils.

(iii) Raised platelet count is present in about half the patients.

(iv) The neutrophil alkaline phosphatase score is usually increased above normal.

(v) Increased serum vitamin B_{12} binding capacity due to an increase in transcobalamin I.

(vi) The bone marrow is hypercellular with prominent megakaryocytes (Fig. 10.2a).

(vii) Blood viscosity increased.

(viii) Plasma urate often increased.

Differential diagnosis

It is essential to exclude other causes of polycythaemia (see Table 10.1). Patients with secondary polycythaemia often have clinical features of the primary diagnosis causing the polycythaemia. Differential diagnosis is usually made as a result of the sequential application of:

(i) TRCV and plasma volume estimation.

(ii) Bone marrow examination.

(iii) Neutrophil alkaline phosphatase and serum vitamin-B_{12} binding protein measurements.

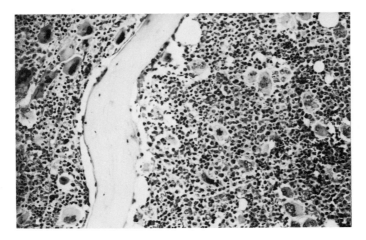

Fig. 10.2a Iliac crest bone marrow trephine biopsy in polycythaemia vera. Fat spaces are replaced by haemopoietic tissue. All haemopoietic cell lines are increased with megakaryocytes particularly prominent.

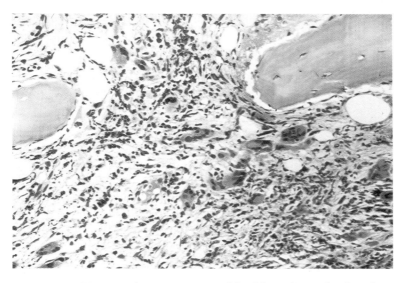

Fig. 10.2b Iliac crest bone marrow trephine biopsy in myelosclerosis (myelofibrosis). Normal marrow architecture is lost and haemopoietic cells are surrounded by increased fibrous tissue and intercellular substance.

(iv) Arterial oxygen estimation (to exclude a cardiac or pulmonary cause).

(v) Haemoglobin electrophoresis and O_2 dissociation studies ($P_{50}O_2$) (to exclude an abnormal haemoglobin).

(vi) Intravenous pyelography (to exclude a kidney lesion).

IVP. ≡ IVU.

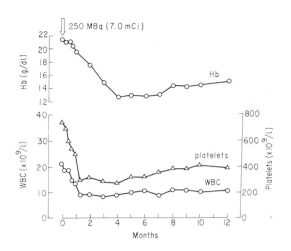

Fig. 10.3 Haematological response to therapy with radioactive phosphorus (^{32}P) in polycythaemia rubra vera.

(vii) <u>Erythropoietin assays</u>. If these are available the results are normal or low in polycythaemia vera, high in secondary polycythaemia and normal in relative polycythaemia.

Therapy

Treatment is aimed at maintaining a normal blood count. The PCV should be less than 50% and preferably around 45% or less.

VENESECTION. This form of therapy is particularly useful when a <u>rapid reduction of red cell volume</u> is required, e.g. at the start of therapy. It is <u>especially indicated in younger patients</u> and those with <u>mild disease</u>. The resulting iron deficiency itself may limit erythropoiesis. Venesection <u>does not control the platelet count</u>.

CYTOTOXIC MYELOSUPPRESSION. <u>Continuous daily or intermittent high dose therapy with bulsulphan or hydroxyurea</u>. This therapy <u>requires close supervision</u> and <u>regular blood counts</u> to prevent overdosage.

PHOSPHORUS-32 (^{32}P) THERAPY. This is <u>excellent</u> therapy for <u>patients with severe disease</u>. ^{32}P is a beta-emitter, with a half-life of 14.3 days. It is <u>concentrated in bone</u> and is a <u>most effective myelosuppressive agent.</u> A typical response to ^{32}P is shown in Fig. 10.3. The usual remission time after a single dose is two years.

Course and prognosis

<u>Thrombosis and haemorrhage are common</u> and <u>vascular accidents are a frequent cause of death</u>. Increased viscosity, vascular stasis,

and high platelet levels may all contribute to thrombosis. Vascular distension, infarcts of small vessels, and defective platelet function may promote haemorrhage. Median survivals with different treatment methods are as follows: venesection alone 4–5 years, chemotherapy 10–16 years, phosphorus-32 10–16 years.

Transition from PV to myelosclerosis occurs in 30% and from PV to acute leukaemia in about 15% of patients. ^{32}P was blamed for the high rate of conversion. Now it is generally accepted that transition is part of the natural history of PV and the high incidence in ^{32}P-treated patients is a result of their longer survival. A similar incidence of leukaemia occurs in patients treated by chemotherapy.

Relative ('stress') polycythaemia

Relative polycythaemia, also known as 'stress' polycythaemia or pseudo-polycythaemia, is the result of plasma volume contraction. The total red cell volume is normal. This condition is more common than polycythaemia vera. It occurs particularly in middle-aged men and may be associated with cardiovascular problems, e.g. myocardial ischaemia or cerebral transient ischaemic attacks. In association with hypertension it has been termed Gaisbock's syndrome. Diuretic therapy and heavy smoking are frequent associations. The value of any particular form of treatment is not decided but trials of repeated venesection with or without plasma replacement are in progress.

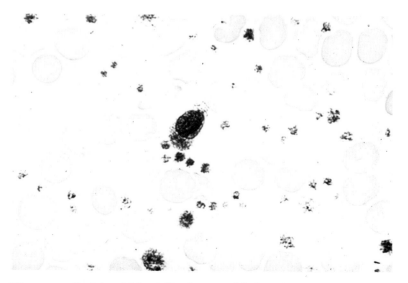

Fig. 10.4 Peripheral blood film in essential thrombocythaemia showing increased numbers of large platelets and a megakaryocytic fragment.

ESSENTIAL THROMBOCYTHAEMIA

Megakaryocyte proliferation and overproduction of platelets is the dominant feature of this condition; there is a sustained increase in platelet count above $1\,000 \times 10^9/l$. The condition is closely related to polycythaemia vera. Some cases show patchy myelosclerosis. Recurrent haemorrhage and thrombosis are the principal clinical features. Splenic enlargement is frequent in the early phase but splenic atrophy due to platelets blocking the splenic microcirculation is seen in many patients.

There may be anaemia (often due to iron deficiency from chronic gastrointestinal haemorrhage) or the thrombocythaemia may be accompanied by polycythaemia.

Laboratory findings, treatment and course

Abnormal large platelets and megakaryocyte fragments may be seen in the blood film (Fig. 10.4). The condition must be distinguished from other causes of a raised platelet count (Table 10.3). Platelet function tests (see p. 221) are consistently abnormal. ^{32}P or alkylating agents are employed to reduce platelet production;

Table 10.3 Causes of a raised platelet count.

Reactive $-600 - 700 \times 10^9 / l$
Haemorrhage, trauma, post-operative
Chronic iron deficiency
Malignancy
Chronic infections
Connective tissue diseases, e.g. rheumatoid arthritis
Post-splenectomy with continuing haemolytic anaemia
Endogenous $> 1,000 \times 10^9 / l$
Essential thrombocythaemia
In some cases of polycythaemia vera, myelosclerosis and chronic granulocytic leukaemia

the doses required are less than in polycythaemia vera. Control of haemorrhage may lead to an increase in TRCV to polycythaemic levels.

MYELOSCLEROSIS (MYELOFIBROSIS)

This condition has many names: (chronic) myelosclerosis, myelofibrosis, agnogenic myeloid metaplasia, or myelofibrosis with myeloid metaplasia (MMM). Haemopoietic stem cell proliferation is more generalised with splenic and hepatic involvement. There is secondary fibrosis in the bone marrow. It is likely that abnormal megakaryocyte precursors release growth factors which stimulate fibroblasts. A third or more of the patients have a previous history

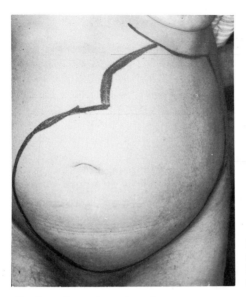

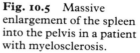

Fig. 10.5 Massive enlargement of the spleen into the pelvis in a patient with myelosclerosis.

of polycythaemia vera and some present with clinical and laboratory features of both disorders ('intermediate myeloproliferative disease').

Clinical features

(i) An insidious onset in older people is usual with symptoms of anaemia.

(ii) Symptoms due to massive splenomegaly (e.g. abdominal dis-

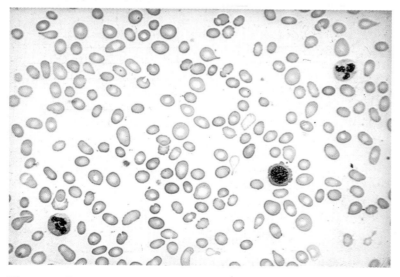

Fig. 10.6 Peripheral blood film in myelosclerosis. There is marked anisocytosis and poikilocytosis with occasional 'tear-drop' cells. The central nucleated cell is an erythroblast.

comfort, pain or indigestion) are frequent; splenomegaly is the main physical finding (Fig. 10.5).

(iii) Loss of weight, anorexia, and night sweats are common.

(iv) Bleeding problems, bone pain or gout occur in a minority of patients.

Myelosclerosis and chronic granulocytic leukaemia are responsible for most cases of massive (>20 cm) splenic enlargement in Britain and North America.

Laboratory investigations

(i) Anaemia is usual but a normal or increased haemoglobin level may be found in patients with intermediate myeloproliferative disease.

(ii) The white cell and platelet counts are frequently high at the time of presentation. Later in the disease leucopenia and thrombocytopenia are common.

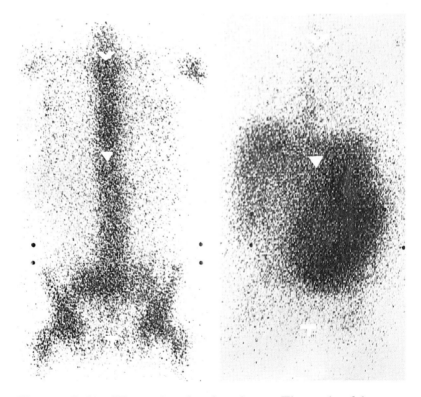

Fig. 10.7 (*Left*) ^{52}Fe scan in polycythaemia vera. The uptake of the isotope in the axial skeleton indicates the sites of bone marrow erythropoiesis. (*Right*) ^{52}Fe scan in myelosclerosis. The heavy concentration of isotope in the splenic and liver areas indicates extramedullary erythropoiesis in these organs.

(iii) A leuco-erythroblastic blood film is found (Fig. 10.6). The red cells show characteristic 'tear-drop' poikilocytes.

(iv) Bone marrow is usually unobtainable by aspiration. Trephine biopsy (see Fig. 10.2b) may show a hypercellular marrow with an increase in reticulin fibre pattern; in other patients there is an increase in intercellular substance and variable collagen deposition. Increased megakaryocytes are frequently seen. In some cases there is an increased bone formation with increased bone density on X-ray.

(v) Low serum folate, raised serum vitamin B_{12} and vitamin B_{12} binding capacity, and an increased neutrophil alkaline phosphatase score are usual.

(vi) High serum urate, LDH and hydroxybutyrate dehydrogenase levels reflect the increased but largely ineffective turnover of haemopoietic cells.

(vii) Extramedullary erythropoiesis may be documented by radio-iron studies (Fig. 10.7) or by liver biopsy.

Therapy

(i) Supportive blood transfusions and regular folic acid therapy are used in anaemic patients.

(ii) Alkylating agents, e.g. busulphan or hydroxyurea, are used in patients with evidence of gross myeloproliferation and hypermetabolism. Allopurinol is needed to prevent urate nephropathy and gout.

(iii) Splenic irradiation may also reduce myeloproliferation temporarily; it reduces splenic size and alleviates symptoms due to hypermetabolism and the enlarged spleen.

(iv) Splenectomy is considered for patients with: **a** unacceptable transfusion requirements; **b** massive splenomegaly causing distressing symptoms which cannot be controlled by radiotherapy or chemotherapy and **c** severe thrombocytopenia which is associated with recurrent haemorrhage. In advanced disease with massive splenomegaly the operative risk is considerable; the patients are in poor general condition and there is a high mortality from postoperative haemorrhage and infection. Post-splenectomy thrombocytosis carries with it a high risk of thromboembolism.

Course and prognosis

The median survival is about 3–4 years but many patients live 10 years or longer. Death is usually from haemorrhage, infection, cardiac or renal failure. Less than 10% of patients develop a terminal blast cell (acute leukaemia) transformation.

ACUTE MYELOSCLEROSIS AND MEGAKARYOBLASTIC LEUKAEMIA

These patients present with a short illness, clinical features due to thrombocytopenia, neutropenia and/or anaemia. There is usually a pancytopenia with occasional abnormal blast cells in the peripheral blood. Attempts at aspirating bone marrow are unsuccessful but trephine biopsy reveals abnormal primitive megakarocytic cells and an increased amount of reticulin fibre. Most cases are now thought to be acute megakaryoblastic leukaemia, but non-Hodgkin's lymphoma and tuberculosis may occasionally give rise to a very similar presentation.

SELECTED BIBLIOGRAPHY

Clinics in Haematology (1975) vol. 4.2, *Polycythaemia and Myelofibrosis.* Ed. A. Videbeck. W.B. Saunders, Philadelphia.
Seminars in Hematology (1975, 1976) vols. 12.4 & 13.1, *Polycythaemia I and II.* Ed. N.I. Berlin. Grune and Stratton, New York.
Major textbooks of haematology (see Chapter 1).

Chapter 11
Platelets, blood coagulation and haemostasis

PLATELETS

Platelet production

Platelets are produced in the bone marrow by fragmentation of the cytoplasm of megakaryocytes. The precursor of the mega-karyocyte—the megakaryoblast—arises by a process of differentiation from the haemopoietic stem cell. The megakaryocyte matures by a process of endomitotic synchronous nuclear replication, enlarging the cytoplasmic volume as the number of nuclei increases in multiples of 2. At a variable stage in development, most commonly at the 8 nucleus stage, further nuclear replication and cell growth ceases, the cytoplasm becomes granular and platelets are then liberated (Fig. 11.1). Platelet production follows the

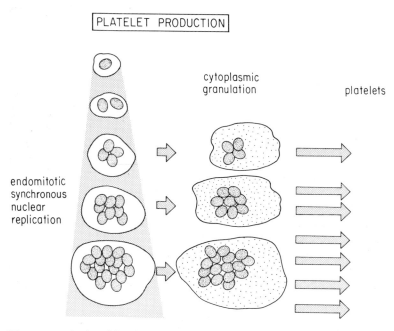

Fig. 11.1 A simplified diagram to illustrate platelet production from megakaryocytes.

formation of microvesicles in the cytoplasm of the cell which co-
alesce to form platelet demarcation membranes. Each megakaryocyte is responsible for the production of about 4000 platelets. The
time interval from differentiation of the stem cell to the production
of platelets averages about 10 days in man.

Platelet production is under the control of a humoral agent
known as thrombopoietin. The nature and site of thrombopoietin
formation have not been established but there is good evidence
that levels are increased in thrombocytopenic patients. Platelet
production may be increased by increasing the number of megakaryocytes and also by increasing the mean volume or nuclear
units of the total megakaryocyte population.

Platelet circulation

Platelets can be labelled in vitro with ^{51}Cr and ^{111}In or in vivo with
DF^{32}P or ^{75}Se-selenomethionine. ^{51}Cr and ^{111}In are the most satisfactory labels for clinical studies. The normal platelet lifespan is 7–
10 days. The normal platelet count is about $250 \times 10^9/l$ (range 150–
$400 \times 10^9/l$). The mean platelet diameter is 1–2 μm and the mean
cell volume 5.8 fl. The volume of platelets diminishes as they
mature in the circulation. Recent evidence suggests that young
platelets may spend up to 24–36 hours in the spleen after being
released from the bone marrow and up to one-third of the marrow
output of platelets may be trapped at any one time in the normal
spleen. Splenic stasis does not normally result in any injury to the
platelet.

Platelet structure

The ultrastructure of platelets is represented in Fig. 11.2. The
mucopolysaccharide surface coat is particularly important in the
platelet reactions of adhesion and aggregation which form the
initial events leading to platelet plug formation during haemostasis. A trilaminar plasma membrane and its open membrane
(canalicular) system invaginates into the platelet interior to form a
large reactive surface to which the plasma coagulation proteins may
be selectively absorbed. These membranes are the structural basis
of platelet factor 3. The contractile thrombasthenin (actomyosin)
system comprises filaments and microfilaments in the sub-mem-
branous area. A circumferential skeleton of microtubules is responsible for the maintenance of the normal circulating discoid shape.
In the platelet interior calcium, nucleotides (particularly ADP),
and serotonin are contained in electron-dense granules. Specific
(alpha) granules contain a heparin antagonist (platelet factor 4),
platelet growth factor, β thromboglobulin, fibrinogen and other
clotting factors. Other specific granules are lysosomes which contain
hydrolytic enzymes. During the release reaction described below,

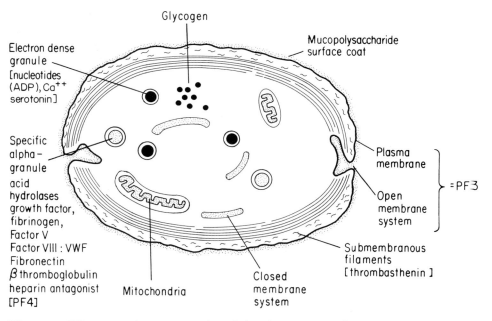

Glycogen

Electron dense
granule
[nucleotides
(ADP),Ca++
serotonin]

Mucopolysaccharide
surface coat

Specific
alpha –
granule
acid
hydrolases
growth factor,
fibrinogen,
Factor V
Factor VIII : VWF
Fibronectin
β thromboglobulin
heparin antagonist
[PF4]

Mitochondria

Closed
membrane
system

Plasma
membrane

Open
membrane
system

⎫
⎬ =PF3
⎭

Submembranous
filaments
[thrombasthenin]

Fig. 11.2 Diagrammatic representation of the ultrastructure of platelets.

the contents of the granules are discharged into the open membrane system. Energy for platelet reactions is derived from oxidative phosphorylation in mitochondria and also from anaerobic glycolysis utilising platelet glycogen. The closed membrane (dense tubular) system of platelets represents residual endoplasmic reticulum.

Platelet function

The main function of platelets is the formation of mechanical plugs during the normal haemostatic response to vascular injury. Central to this function are the platelet reactions of adhesion, release, aggregation and fusion as well as their procoagulant activity.

PLATELET ADHESION. Following blood vessel injury, platelets adhere to the exposed subendothelial connective tissues. This vital function is dependent upon a part of the factor VIII protein in plasma known as the von Willebrand factor which is part of the main fraction of the factor VIII molecule, factor VIIIR:AG (factor VIII-related antigen) (Fig. 11.3). The relationship of this part of factor VIII to the coagulation active molecule is described later in this chapter. Adhesion is also dependent on a platelet surface membrane glycoprotein which is absent in the rare Bernard-Soulier syndrome (see p. 220).

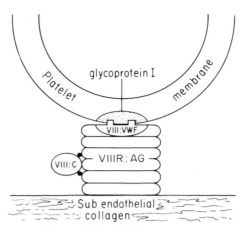

Fig. 11.3 The role of factor VIII:VWF and factor VIIIR:AG in platelet adhesion.

THE RELEASE REACTION. Collagen exposure or thrombin action results in the release of platelet granule contents which include ADP, serotonin, fibrinogen, lysosomal enzymes and heparin neutralising factor (platelet factor 4). Collagen and thrombin activate platelet prostaglandin synthesis (Fig. 11.4)

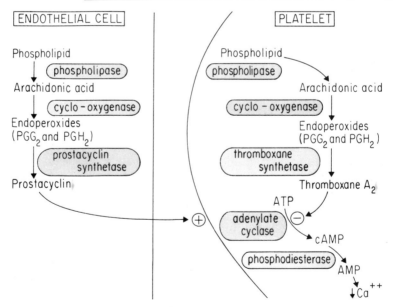

Fig. 11.4 The synthesis of prostacylin and thromboxane. The opposing effects of these agents are mediated by changes in concentration of cyclic AMP in platelets via stimulation or inhibition of the enzyme adenylate cyclase. Cyclic AMP controls the concentration of free calcium ions in the platelet which are important in the processes which cause adhesion and aggregation. High levels of cyclic AMP lead to low free calcium ion concentrations and prevent aggregation and adhesion.

leading to the formation of a labile substance, thromboxane A$_2$, $\rightarrow \uparrow$ surface Ca^{2+} which lowers platelet cyclic AMP levels and initiates the release reaction. This substance not only potentiates platelet aggregation but also has powerful vasoconstrictive activity. The release re-action is inhibited by substances which increase the level of platelet cyclic AMP. One such substance is the prostaglandin prostacyclin (PGI$_2$) which is synthesised by vascular endothelial cells. It is a potent inhibitor of platelet aggregation and probably prevents their deposition on normal vascular endothelium.

PLATELET AGGREGATION. Released ADP and thromboxane A$_2$ cause additional platelets to aggregate at the site of vascular injury. ADP causes platelets to swell and encourages the platelet membranes of adjacent platelets to adhere to each other. As they do so further release reactions occur liberating more ADP and thromboxane A$_2$ causing secondary platelet aggregation. This self-perpetuating process of platelet aggregation results in the formation of a platelet mass large enough to plug the area of endothelial injury.

PLATELET PROCOAGULANT ACTIVITY. After platelet aggregation and release the exposed membrane phospholipid (platelet factor 3) is available for coagulation protein complex formation. This phospholipid surface forms an ideal template for the crucial concentration and orientation of these proteins for the normal coagulation cascade reactions (Fig. 11.5).

PLATELET FUSION. High concentrations of ADP, the enzymes released during the release reaction and thrombasthenin contri-bute to an irreversible fusion of platelets aggregated at the site of vascular injury. Thrombin also encourages fusion of platelets, and fibrin formation reinforces the stability of the evolving platelet plug.

The growth factor found in the specific granules of platelets stimulates vascular smooth muscle cells to multiply and this may hasten vascular healing following injury.

BLOOD COAGULATION

Blood coagulation involves a biological amplification system in which relatively few initiation substances sequentially activate by proteolysis a cascade of circulating precursor proteins (the coagu-lation factor enzymes) which culminate in the generation of throm-bin; this, in turn, converts soluble plasma fibrinogen into fibrin (Fig. 11.5). Fibrin enmeshes the platelet aggregates at the sites of vascular injury and converts the rather unstable primary platelet plugs to firm, definitive and stable haemostatic plugs. A list of the coagulation factors appears in Table 11.1.

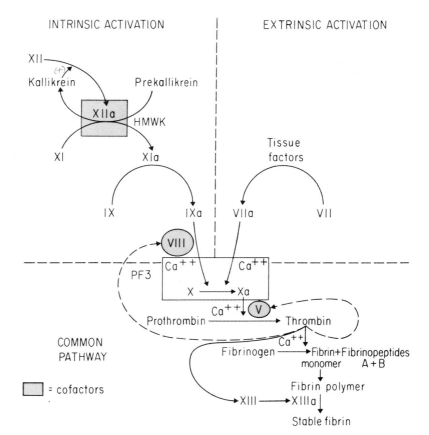

INTRINSIC ACTIVATION | EXTRINSIC ACTIVATION

Fig. 11.5 The pathways of blood coagulation.

The operation of this enzyme cascade requires local concentration of circulating coagulation factors at the site of injury. Surface-mediated reactions occur on exposed collagen, platelet factor 3 and tissue factors. With the exception of fibrinogen, which is the fibrin clot subunit, the coagulation factors are either enzyme precursors or cofactors (see Table 11.1). All the enzymes, except factor XIII are serine proteases, i.e. their ability to hydrolyse peptide bonds depends upon the amino-acid serine at their active centre (Fig. 11.6). The scale of amplication achieved in this system is dramatic, e.g. one mole of activated factor XI through sequential activation of factors IX, X and prothrombin may generate up to 2×10^8 moles of fibrin.

In the *intrinsic system*, exposed collagen and other negatively charged components of subendothelial connective tissue cause activation of factor XII. This activates factor XI and also converts prekallikrein to kallikrein. Kallikrein and factor XI are bound to a cofactor, high-molecular-weight kininogen (HMWK). During this

Table 11.1   The coagulation factors.

Roman numeral	Descriptive name	Active form
I	Fibrinogen	Fibrin subunit
II	Prothrombin	Serine protease
III	Tissue factor	
IV	Calcium ions	
V	Proaccelerin	Cofactor
VII	Proconvertin	Serine protease
VIII	Antihaemophilic factor/von Willebrand factor	Cofactor
IX	Christmas factor (plasma thromboplastin component)	Serine protease
X	Stuart-Prower factor	Serine protease
XI	Plasma thromboplastin antecedent	Serine protease
XII	Hageman (contact) factor	Serine protease
XIII	Fibrin stabilising factor	Transglutaminase
—	Prekallikrein (Fletcher factor)	Serine protease
—	HMW kininogen (Fitzgerald factor)	Cofactor

Note   The descriptive names fibrinogen, prothrombin, tissue factor, and calcium are used in preference to the roman numeral. Factor VI originally referred to activated factor V and has now been abandoned. The nomenclature for the kinin system was developed before it was known that prekallikrein and HMW kininogen also had a role in the coagulation system.

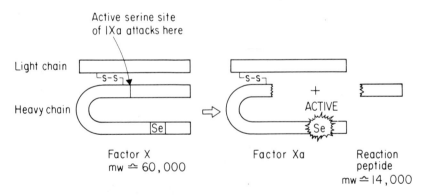

Fig. 11.6   Serine protease activity. This example shows the activation of factor X by factor IX. Se = serine.

contact phase of coagulation activation, kallikrein cleaves the small vasoactive peptide bradykinin from HMWK. In addition, kallikrein has an autocatalytic effect on coagulation by causing further activation of factor XII.

The next reaction in the enzyme sequence of the intrinsic system involves the activation of factor IX by activated factor XI. In association with calcium and the cofactor factor VIII, activated factor IX then activates factor X on the membrane surface provided by platelet factor 3.

In the *extrinsic pathway*, tissue factors (lipoproteins from damaged cells) activate coagulation factor VII which in turn activates factor X directly.

In the *final common pathway*, activated factor X in association with cofactor factor V, calcium and platelet factor 3 converts prothrombin into thrombin. Thrombin hydrolyses arginine–lysine bonds of fibrinogen releasing fibrinopeptides A and B to form fibrin monomer (Fig. 11.8). Fibrin monomers link spontaneously by hydrogen bonds to form a loose, insoluble fibrin polymer. Factor XIII activated by thrombin and calcium stabilises the fibrin polymers with the formation of covalent bond cross-links.

The extrinsic and intrinsic systems complement each other. It is likely that, following tissue injury, the tissue activators produce small amounts of thrombin which, in addition to producing fibrin, will greatly accelerate the intrinsic pathway by activation of the cofactors factor VIII and factor V. Because patients with a deficiency of factors in either system may suffer from severe bleeding problems it is obvious that both are required for normal haemostasis.

Some of the properties of the coagulation factors are listed in Table 11.2. The activity of factors II, VII, IX and X is dependent upon vitamin K which is responsible for a post-ribosomal γ carboxylation of a number of terminal glutamic acid residues on each of these molecules. The carboxylation facilitates the binding of calcium required to form complexes with phospholipid (Fig. 11.7). In the absence of vitamin K no carboxylation of glutamic acid residues occurs, calcium is not bound and these factors are not linked to platelet phospholipid. Without the critical concentration and orientation of these reacting coagulation factors the rate of prothrombin conversion to thrombin is minimal.

Table 11.2 The coagulation factors.

Fibrinogen Group: Factors I, V, VIII, XIII
  Thrombin interacts with them all
  Activity lost in coagulation process (not present in serum)
  Increase during inflammation, in pregnancy and women on oral contraceptives
  V and VIII lose activity in stored plasma

Prothrombin Group: Factors II, VII, IX, X
  Dependent on vitamin K for synthesis, require Ca^{++} for activation
  All except prothrombin (II) are not consumed during coagulation (present in serum)
  Stable, well preserved in stored plasma

Contact Group: Factors XI, XII, prekallikrein
  Not dependent on vitamin K for synthesis, not calcium dependent
  Stable, well preserved in stored plasma

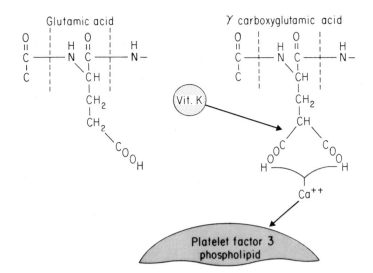

Fig. 11.7 The action of vitamin K in γ carboxylation of glutamic acid in factors II, VII, IX and X which are then able to bind Ca^{++} and bind to platelet factor 3 phospholipid.

Factor VIII is a large protein (mol. wt. $1.5–2.0 \times 10^6$) which contains two functional entities. The major bulk of the protein which precipitates with heterologous antisera, factor VIII-related antigen (VIIIR:AG), is associated with platelet-related activities such as their adhesion to exposed subendothelial connective tissues and ristocetin-induced aggregation. Von Willebrand's factor (VIII:WF) is the part of factor VIIIR:AG which is involved in these activities. This protein circulates as a complex molecule comprised of several subunit-chains of similar size which are linked by disulphide bonds. The molecular weight of the multimers varies from 800 000 to 12 000 000. The smaller entity associated with coagulant activity (VIII:C) is linked to the VIIIR:AG molecule by non-covalent bonds (see Fig. 11.3). The synthesis of VIIIR:AG occurs in endothelial cells. This entity either combines with VIII:C or is somehow altered to acquire this activity. Whether this takes place in the endothelial cells or whether the VIIIR:AG protein circulates to another site, e.g. liver or spleen, where it is joined to or activated to VIII:C is unknown.

Factor VIII:C, like factor V, is a cofactor which requires modification by a serine protease, usually thrombin, to become fully active.

Factor VIII is associated with the marginal circulation and vascular endothelium. The stress of exercise or infusion of either adrenaline or desmopressin (DDAVP) produces considerable increase in the level of circulating factor VIII. Following its modification by thrombin or other serine proteases, factor VIII activity is unstable. In blood stored at 4°C for transfusion there is a progressive fall in activity to less than 10% during the first three days.

Fibrinogen has a mol. wt. of 340 000 and consists of three pairs of polypeptide chains αA, βB; and γ which are linked by disulphide bonds (Fig. 11.8). After cleavage of fibrinopeptides A + B, fibrin monomer consists of three paired α, β, and γ chains.

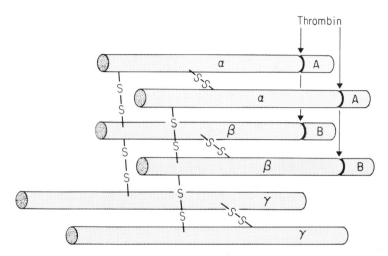

Fig. 11.8 The structure of fibrinogen and sites of action of thrombin in releasing fibrinopeptides A and B from fibrinogen.

Physiological limitation of blood coagulation

Unchecked blood coagulation would lead to dangerous occlusion of blood vessels (thrombosis) if the following protective mechanisms were not in operation.

1. PLASMA INHIBITORS OF ACTIVATED FACTORS. It is important that the effect of thrombin is limited to the site of injury. There is direct inactivation of thrombin (and other serine protease factors) by circulating inhibitors. Antithrombin III is the most potent of these. It inactivates serine proteases by combining with them by peptide bonding to form high-molecular-weight stable complexes. Heparin potentiates its action markedly. α_2-macroglobulins, α_2-antiplasmin and α_2-antitrypsin also exert an inhibitory effect on circulating serine proteases. The complement system C_1 esterase inhibitor is a potent inhibitor of plasma kallkrein.

Thrombin binds to an endothelial cell surface receptor known as thrombomodulin. It has been established recently that the resulting complex activates a circulating vitamin K-dependent precursor of the serine proteases known as protein C. This protein is able to destroy factors V and VIII, thus preventing further thrombin generation.

2. BLOOD FLOW. At the periphery of a damaged area of tissue, blood flow rapidly achieves a dilution and dispersal of activated factors before fibrin formation has occurred. Activated factors are destroyed by liver parenchymal cells and particulate matter is removed by liver Kupffer cells and other RE cells.

3. PLASMIN AND FIBRIN SPLIT PRODUCTS. Plasmin generation (see below) at the site of injury also limits the extent of the evolving thrombus by digesting fibrin, fibrinogen and factors V and VIII. The split products of fibrinolysis are competitive inhibitors of thrombin and fibrin polymerisation.

FIBRINOLYSIS

Fibrinolysis (like coagulation) is a normal haemostatic response to vascular injury. Plasminogen, a beta globulin pro-enzyme in blood and tissue fluid, is converted to the serine protease, plasmin by activators either from the vessel wall (intrinsic activation) or from the tissues (extrinsic activation) (Fig. 11.9). Release of circulating plasminogen-activator from endothelial cells occurs after such stimuli as trauma, exercise or emotional stress. Activated factor XII also potentiates the action of plasminogen activator. The fibrinolytic agent, streptokinase, is a peptide produced by β haemolytic streptococci. It forms a complex with plasminogen, which activates other plasminogen molecules.

Plasmin has a wider range of activity than thrombin, hydrolysing

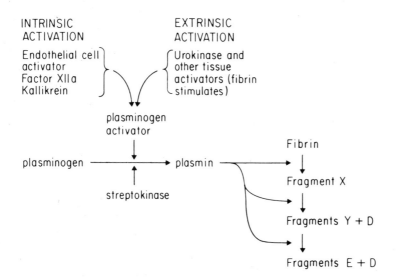

Fig. 11.9 The fibrinolytic system.

both arginine and lysine peptide bonds. It is capable of digesting fibrinogen, fibrin, factors V and VIII and many other proteins. Cleavage of peptide bonds in fibrin and fibrinogen produces a variety of split (degradation) products (FDPs) (see Fig. 11.9). The largest split product, fragment X, which is released from early digestion of fibrinogen or fibrin, retains thrombin-susceptible sites and thus is a competitive inhibitor of thrombin. A later and smaller digestion fragment, Y, is a competitive inhibitor of fibrin polymerisation. Large amounts of the smallest fragments D and E are detected in the plasma of patients with disseminated intravascular coagulation.

Inactivation of plasmin

Circulating plasmin is inactivated by potent inhibitors α_2-antiplasmin and α_2-macroglobulin. This prevents widespread destruction of fibrinogen and other coagulation factor proteins.

THE KININ SYSTEM

During the contact phase of coagulation, factor XIIa converts prekallikrein to kallikrein. The large cofactor which binds these two enzymes, high-molecular-weight kininogen, includes a small (nine amino-acid) peptide, bradykinin. This is released after specific proteolytic cleavage by kallikrein.

Bradykinin increases vascular permeability and is a vasodilator. Kallikrein has chemotactic activity for both neutrophils and monocytes and attracts these phagocyte cells to sites of injury or infection.

Factor XII and its associated precursor enzymes thus provide an important link between the homeostatic functions of coagulation, fibrinolysis and inflammation (Fig. 11.10).

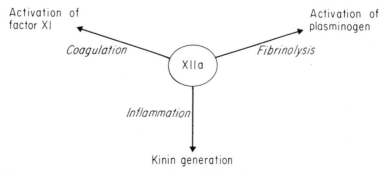

Fig. 11.10 The central role of factor XII in the initial reactions of coagulation, fibrinolysis and inflammation.

THE ENDOTHELIAL CELL

The role of the endothelial cell in the maintenance of vascular integrity is well established. This cell provides the basement membrane, collagen, elastin and fibrinectin of the subendothelial connective tissue. Loss or damage to the endothelial lining results in both haemorrhage and activation of the haemostatic mechanism. The endothelial cell also has an active role in the haemostatic response. Synthesis of prostacyclin, factors VIIIR:AG and VIII:VWF, plasminogen activator, antithrombin III and thrombomodulin, the surface protein responsible for activation of protein C provides agents which are vital to both platelet reactions and blood coagulation (Fig. 11.11). There is also evidence that endothelial cells, especially in the pulmonary microcirculation, remove potential vasoactive and platelet aggregating agents such as serotonin, bradykinin and angiotensin I from the circulating blood.

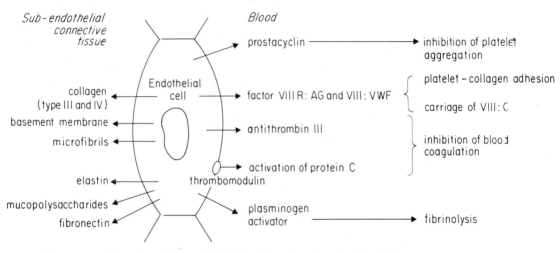

Fig. 11.11   The role of the endothelial cell in protecting the blood from coagulation and platelets from subendothelial aggregating substances.

THE HAEMOSTATIC RESPONSE

The normal haemostatic response to vascular damage depends on closely linked interaction between the blood vessel wall, circulating platelets and blood coagulation factors (Fig. 11.12).

Vasoconstriction

An immediate vasoconstriction of the injured vessel and reflex constriction of adjacent small arteries and arterioles is responsible for an initial slowing of blood flow to the area of injury. When there is widespread damage this vascular reaction prevents exsanguination. The reduced blood flow allows contact activation of platelets and coagulation factors. The vasoactive amines and thromboxane from platelets, and the fibrinopeptides liberated during fibrin formation, also have vasoconstrictive activity.

Platelet reactions and primary haemostatic plug formation

Following a break in the endothelial lining, there is an initial adherence of platelets to exposed connective tissue (Fig. 11.12). This platelet adhesion is potentiated by a portion of the factor VIII protein, von Willebrand's factor. Collagen exposure and thrombin produced at the site of injury cause the adherent platelets to release their granule contents which include ADP, serotonin, fibrinogen, lysosomal enzymes and heparin neutralising factor. Collagen and thrombin activate platelet prostaglandin synthesis leading to the formation of thromboxane A_2 which potentiates platelet release reactions, platelet aggregation and also has powerful vasoconstrictive activity. Released ADP causes platelets to swell and aggregate. Additional platelets from the circulating blood are drawn to the area of injury. This self-perpetuating platelet aggregation promotes the growth of the haemostatic plug which soon covers the exposed

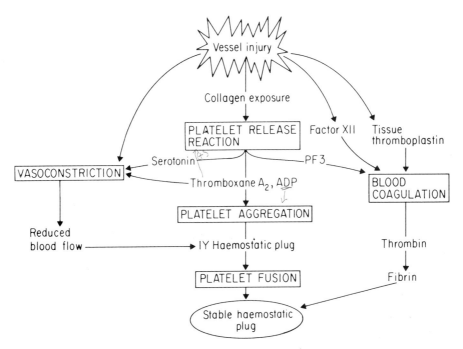

Fig. 11.12 Reactions involved in haemostasis.

connective tissue. Released platelet granule enzymes, ADP and thrombasthenin may all contribute to the fusion of the accumulated platelets. It seems likely that prostacyclin produced by endothelial and smooth muscle cells in the vessel wall adjacent to the area of damage is important in limiting the extent of the initial platelet plug. The rather unstable primary haemostatic plug produced by these platelet reactions in the first minute or so following injury is usually sufficient to provide temporary control of bleeding.

Definitive haemostasis is achieved when fibrin formed by blood coagulation is added to the platelet mass.

Stabilisation of platelet plug by fibrin

Following vascular injury, activation of both coagulation pathways occurs — factor XII of the intrinsic pathway is activated by exposed collagen, while leakage of tissue factors activates factor VII of the extrinsic system. Platelet aggregation and release reactions accelerate the coagulation process by providing abundant membrane lipoprotein PF3. Thrombin generated at the injury site converts soluble plasma fibrinogen into fibrin and also potentiates platelet aggregation and release reactions. A meshwork of fibrin anchors and extends the platelet plug. The fibrin component of the haemostatic plug increases as the fused platelets autolyse and after 24–28 hours the entire haemostatic plug is transformed into a solid mass of fibrin.

TESTS OF HAEMOSTATIC FUNCTION

Defective haemostasis with abnormal bleeding may result from thrombocytopenia, a disorder of platelet function or defective blood coagulation. Patients with a number of vascular disorders may also suffer from a bleeding disorder. A number of simple tests are employed to assess the platelet and coagulation components of haemostasis.

Blood count and blood film examination

As thrombocytopenia is the commonest cause of abnormal bleeding, patients with suspected bleeding disorders should initially have a blood count including platelet count and blood film examination. In addition to establishing the presence of thrombocytopenia, the cause of this may be obvious, e.g. an acute leukaemia.

Bleeding time

When the blood count, platelet count and film examination are normal the bleeding time is done to detect abnormal platelet function. This test measures platelet plug formation *in vivo*. In the Ivy template method, after the application of 40 mmHg pressure to the upper arm with a blood pressure cuff, two 1 mm deep, 1 cm long incisions are made in the flexor surface forearm skin. Bleeding stops normally in 3–8 minutes and there is a progressive prolongation with platelet counts less than $75 \times 10^9/l$. Long times are found in patients with disorders of platelet function and in some patients with intrinsic vascular disorders.

Screening tests of blood coagulation

Screening tests may provide an assessment of the extrinsic and intrinsic systems of blood coagulation and also the central conversion of fibrinogen to fibrin (Table 11.3). In general, prolongation of clotting times beyond those of normal 'control' plasmas in the test system will indicate a deficiency.

1   THE PROTHROMBIN TIME (PT) measures the extrinsic system (factor VII) as well as factors common to both systems (factors X, V, prothrombin and fibrinogen). Tissue thromboplastin (brain extract) and calcium are added to plasma. The normal time for clotting is 10–14 seconds.

Table 11.3   Laboratory tests used in the diagnosis of coagulation disorders.

SCREENING TESTS	Function	Normal clotting time
Prothrombin time (PT)	Tests extrinsic and common pathways	10–14 sec.
Activated partial thromboplastin time (APTT or PTTK)	Tests intrinsic and common pathways	30–40 sec.
Thrombin time (TT)	Tests fibrinogen–fibrin conversion	10–12 sec.

SPECIFIC ASSAYS
   Most are based on an APTT or PT in which all factors except the one to be measured are present in the substrate plasma. The corrective effect of an unknown plasma on the prolonged time of the deficient plasma is compared with the corrective effect of normal plasma. Results are expressed as percentage of normal activity.

TESTS OF FIBRINOLYSIS
Euglobulin clot lysis time, tests for fibrin degradation products (FDPs).

2 THE ACTIVATED PARTIAL THROMBOPLASTIN TIME (APTT) measures the intrinsic system factors VIII, IX, XI and XII in addition to factors common to both systems. Three substances — phospholipid, a surface activator (e.g. kaolin), and calcium — are added to plasma. The normal time for clotting is about 30–40 seconds.

Prolonged clotting times in the PT and APTT due to factor deficiency are corrected by the addition of normal plasma to the test plasma. If there is no correction or incomplete correction with normal plasma an inhibitor of coagulation is suspected.

3 SCREENING TESTS FOR FIBRINOGEN DEFICIENCY include fibrinogen titre and thrombin time. These tests are sensitive to the presence of either heparin or fibrin degradation products.

4 THE WHOLE BLOOD COAGULATION TIME AT 37°C is still used by some laboratories. It is generally prolonged only in severe deficiencies. The test may be coupled with observation of clot retraction and clot size at 1 hour.

Specific assays of coagulation factors

Most factor assays are based on an APTT or PT in which all factors except the one to be measured are present in the substrate plasma. This usually requires a supply of plasma from patients with hereditary deficiency of the factor in question. The corrective effect of the unknown plasma on the prolonged clotting time of the deficient substrate plasma is then compared with the corrective effect of normal plasma. Results are expressed as percentage of normal activity. A number of chemical and immunological methods are available for quantitation of plasma fibrinogen, and immune assays have been developed to measure other coagulation factors, particularly factor VIIIR:Ag and factor VIII:C.

Tests of fibrinolysis

Increased levels of circulating plasminogen activator may be detected by demonstrating shortened euglobulin clot lysis times. A number of immunological methods are available to detect fibrinogen or fibrin degradation products (FDPs) in serum. In patients with enhanced fibrinolysis, low levels of circulating plasminogen may be detected.

SELECTED BIBLIOGRAPHY

Bloom A.L. & Thomas D.P. (eds.) (1981) *Haemostasis and Thrombosis*. Churchill Livingstone, Edinburgh.

British Medical Bulletin (1977) **33,** no. 3, *Haemostasis*. Ed. D.P. Thomas.

British Medical Bulletin (1978) **34,** no. 2, *Thrombosis*. Ed. D.P. Thomas.

Clinics in Haematology (1981) vol. 10.2, *Thrombosis*. Ed. C.R.M. Prentice. W.B. Saunders, Philadelphia.

Clinics in Haematology (1983) vol. 12.1, *Platelet Disorders*. Eds. L.A. Harker & T.S. Zimmerman. W.B. Saunders, Philadelphia.

Coleman R.W. *et al* (eds.) (1982) *Hemostasis and Thrombosis: Basic Principles and Clinical Practice*. J.B. Lippincott, Philadelphia.

Esnouff M.P. (1981) Biochemistry of coagulation. In *Recent Advances in Haematology 3*, ed. A.V. Hoffbrand. Churchill Livingstone, Edinburgh.

Gordon J.L. (ed.) (1976) *Platelets in Biology and Pathology*. North Holland, Amsterdam.

Ingram G.I.C., Brozovic M. & Slater M.P.G. (1983) *Bleeding disorders— Investigation and Management*, 2nd edition. Blackwell Scientific Publications, Oxford.

Mann K.G. & Fass D.N. (1982) The molecular biology of blood coagulation. In *Current Hematology 2*, ed. V.F. Fairbanks. Wiley Medical, New York.

Ogston D. (1983) *The Physiology of Hemostasis*. Croom Helm, London.

Progress in Hemostasis and Thrombosis (1982) Vol. 6, Ed. H. Spaet. Grune & Stratton, New York.

Seminars in Hematology (1977) vol 14, no. 3, *Hemostasis and Thrombosis*. Ed. R.S. Mibasham. Grune and Stratton, New York.

Thompson A.R. & Harker L.A. (1983) *Manual of Hemostasis and Thrombosis*, 3rd edition. F.A. Davis, Philadelphia.

Zimmerman T.S. *et al* (1983) Factor VIII/von Willebrand factor. *Progress in Hematology*, *XIII*, 279-310. Ed. E.B. Brown. Grune and Stratton, New York.

Major textbooks of haematology (see Chapter 1).

Chapter 12
Bleeding disorders due to vascular and platelet abnormalities

[handwritten: Bleeding]

[handwritten: 1. Vascular ab⊕]
[handwritten: 2. Platelet ab⊕ < no. function]
[handwritten: 3. Clotting ab⊕]

Abnormal bleeding may result from vascular disorders, thrombocytopenia, platelet function defects or defective coagulation. The first three categories are discussed in this chapter and the disorders of blood coagulation follow in Chapter 13.

VASCULAR BLEEDING DISORDERS

The vascular disorders are a heterogenous group of conditions characterised by easy bruising and spontaneous bleeding from the small vessels. The underlying abnormality is either in the vessels themselves or in the perivascular connective tissues. Most cases of bleeding due to vascular defects alone are not severe. Frequently the bleeding is mainly in the skin causing petechiae, ecchymoses, or both. In some disorders there is also bleeding from mucous membranes. In some of these conditions the standard screening tests show little or no abnormality. The bleeding time is rarely prolonged and the other tests of haemostasis are normal. Vascular defects may be inherited or acquired.

Hereditary haemorrhagic telangiectasia

In this uncommon disorder which is transmitted as an autosomal dominant trait; there are dilated microvascular swellings which appear during childhood and become more numerous in adult life. These telangiectasia develop in the skin, mucous membranes (Fig. 12.1) and internal organs. Recurrent gastrointestinal tract haemorrhage may cause chronic iron deficiency anaemia.

[handwritten: Back of Hands, face.]
[handwritten: Aneurysms : Arch Ao, Renal A.]
[handwritten: A-V. Fistulae]

Acquired vascular defects

Vascular defects from many disorders may result in abnormal bleeding.
1 *Simple easy bruising* is a common benign disorder which occurs in otherwise healthy women, especially those of childbearing age.
2 *Senile purpura* due to atrophy of the supporting tissues of

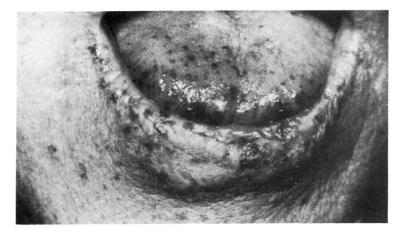

Fig. 12.1 Typical appearance of the lips and tongue in a patient with hereditary capillary telangiectasia.

cutaneous blood vessels is seen mainly on dorsal aspects of the forearm and hand.

3 *Purpura associated with infections* may result from toxic damage to the endothelium, or disseminated intravascular coagulation (see p. 218).

4 *The Henoch–Schönlein syndrome*, an immune complex (Type III) hypersensitivity reaction usually found in children, often follows an acute infection. The characteristic purpuric rash accompanied by localised oedema and itching is often most prominent on the buttocks and extensor surfaces of the lower legs and elbows. Painful joint swelling, haematuria and abdominal pain may also occur. It is usually a self-limiting condition but occasional patients develop renal failure.

5 *Scurvy*. In vitamin C deficiency, defective intercellular substance may cause perifollicular petechiae, bruising and mucosal haemorrhage.

6 *Steroid purpura*. The purpura which is associated with long-term steroid therapy or Cushing's syndrome is caused by defective vascular supportive tissue.

THROMBOCYTOPENIA

Abnormal bleeding associated with thrombocytopenia or abnormal platelet function is also characterised by spontaneous skin purpura and mucosal haemorrhage and prolonged bleeding after trauma. The main causes of thrombocytopenia are listed in Table 12.1.

Bleeding disorders due to vascular and platelet abnormalities   213

Table 12.1   Causes of thrombocytopenia.

Failure of platelet production
Selective megakaryocyte depression
  Drugs, chemicals, viral infections
Part of general bone marrow failure
  Aplastic anaemia
  Leukaemia
  Myelodysplastic syndromes
  Myelosclerosis
  Marow infiltration: e.g. carcinoma, lymphoma
  Multiple myeloma
  Megaloblastic anaemia

Increased destruction of platelets
  Auto-immune thrombocytopenic purpura: chronic, acute
  Secondary immune thrombocytopenia (post-infection, SLE,
  CLL and lymphomas)
  Post-transfusion purpura
  Drug-induced immune thrombocytopenia
  Heparin
  Disseminated intravascular coagulation

Abnormal distribution of platelets
  Splenomegaly

Dilutional loss
  Massive transfusion of old blood to bleeding patients

Platelet production failure

This is the commonest cause of thrombocytopenia. Selective megakaryocyte depression may result from drug toxicity (e.g. phenylbutazone, cotrimoxazole, gold salts, thiazide diuretics, tolbutamide) or from viral infections. Decreased numbers of megakaryocytes may be part of a generalised bone marrow failure in aplastic anaemia, leukaemia, myelosclerosis or marrow infiltrations. Ineffective platelet production from normal or increased numbers of megakaryocytes is a feature of megaloblastic anaemias. Diagnosis of these causes of thrombocytopenia is made from the peripheral blood count, the blood film and bone marrow examination.

Increased destruction of platelets

CHRONIC IMMUNE THROMBOCYTOPENIC PURPURA (ITP)

This is a relatively common disorder with a highest incidence in women aged 15–50. It is usually idiopathic but may be seen in association with other diseases, e.g. SLE, chronic lymphocytic leukaemia, Hodgkin's disease, auto-immune haemolytic anaemia.

PATHOGENESIS. Platelet sensitisation with auto-antibodies (usually IgG) results in their premature removal from the circulation by cells of the reticulo-endothelial system (Fig. 12.2). Lightly sensitised platelets are mainly destroyed in the spleen but heavily sensitised platelets or platelets coated with complement as well as IgG are destroyed throughout the reticulo-endothelial system, mainly in the liver.

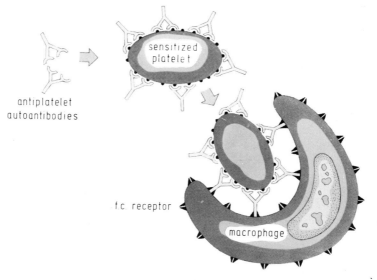

Fig. 12.2 The pathogenesis of thrombocytopenia in chronic immune thrombocytopenic purpura (ITP).

CLINICAL FEATURES. The onset is often insidious with petechial haemorrhage, easy bruising and, in women, menorrhagia. Mucosal bleeding occurs in severe cases but intracranial haemorrhage is rare. The severity of bleeding in ITP is less than that seen in patients with comparable degrees of thrombocytopenia from bone marrow failure; this is attributed to the circulation of predominantly young, functionally superior platelets in ITP.

The spleen is palpable in only 10% of cases.

DIAGNOSIS

(i) The platelet count is usually 10–50 · 10^9/l.

(ii) The blood film shows reduced numbers of platelets, those present often being large.

(iii) The bone marrow shows increased numbers of megakaryocytes.

(iv) Sensitive tests are able to demonstrate antiplatelet IgG either alone or with complement, on the platelet surface or in the serum in most patients.

(v) Autologous platelet survival studies with ^{51}Cr- or ^{111}In-labelled platelets may be used to document reduced platelet survival. In severe cases the mean survival may be reduced to less than one hour.

MANAGEMENT. A spontaneous recovery occurs in less than 10% of patients with chronic ITP. Treatment is aimed at reducing the level of auto-antibody and reducing the destruction rate of sensitised platelets. A proportion of cases relapse, however, months or years after remitting with the treatment discussed below.

1   *Steroids.* 80% of patients remit on high dose corticosteroid therapy. Prednisolone 60 mg daily is the usual initial therapy and the dose is gradually reduced after a remission has been achieved. In poor responders the dose is reduced more slowly but splenectomy or immunosuppression is considered.

2   *Splenectomy* (Fig. 12.3). This operation is recommended in patients who do not recover within three months of steroid therapy or who require unacceptably high doses of steroids to maintain a platelet count above $50 \times 10^9/$l. Good results occur in most of the patients.

3   *Immunosuppressive drugs*, e.g. vincristine, vinblastine, cyclo-

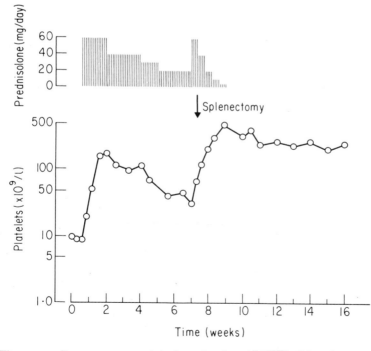

Fig. 12.3 Response to prednisolone in chronic ITP with subsequent relapse and response to splenectomy.

phosphamide, azathioprine, are usually reserved for those patients who do not respond to steriods and splenectomy.

4 *Androgens* (non-virilising). Danazol has been recommended recently, in patients with thrombocytopenia which is unresponsive to corticosteroids and/or splenectomy.

5 *High dose immunoglobulin* has also recently been shown to produce temporary rises in platelet counts. The mechanism may be blockage of Fc receptors on macrophages. The long-term benefits of this approach are unknown.

6 *Platelet transfusions.* Although isologous platelets seldom survive longer than the patient's own, platelet concentrates are beneficial in patients with acute, life-threatening bleeding.

Acute immune thrombocytopenia

also could – get Acute post-infectious Encephalitis

Acute thrombocytopenia is most common in children. The mechanism is not well established. In about 75% of patients, the thrombocytopenia and bleeding follows vaccination or an infection, e.g. measles, chicken pox or infectious mononucleosis and an allergic reaction with immune complex formation and complement deposition on platelets is suspected.

Spontaneous remissions are usual but, in 5–10% of cases, the disease becomes chronic. Short-term steroid therapy is sometimes used in severe cases.

Thrombocytopenia occurring about 10 days after a blood transfusion has been attributed to antibodies in the recipient developing against the Pl^{A1} antigen on transfused platelets. The reason why the patient's own platelets are destroyed is unknown. An immune mechanism also seems likely in patients who develop thrombocytopenia during heparin therapy.

Drug-induced immune thrombocytopenia

An allergic mechanism has been demonstrated as the cause of many drug-induced thrombocytopenias. Drug-induced antibodies have been demonstrated in patients suffering from thrombocytopenia in association with therapy involving quinine (tonic water), quinidine, PAS, sulphonamides, rifampicin, stibophen, digitoxin and other drugs. In most drug-dependent immune thrombocytopenias, the antibody is directed against a drug-plasma protein antigen and circulating immune complexes are adsorbed onto the platelet (Fig. 12.4). The platelet is damaged as an 'innocent bystander' and is removed by the RE cells due to the immunoglobulin or complement coating. If the complement sequence is fully activated, the platelets are lysed directly in the circulation. Patients present with acute purpura sometimes heralded by a chill, headache and flushing.

The platelet count is often less than $10 \times 10^9/l$, and the bone

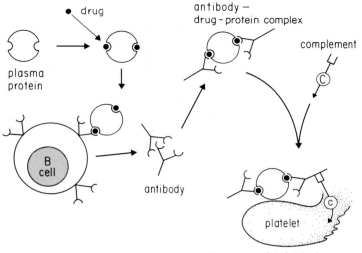

Fig. 12.4 Usual type of platelet damage caused by drugs in which a drug–protein–antibody complex is deposited on the platelet surface. If complement is attached and the sequence goes to completion, the platelet may be lysed directly. Otherwise it is removed by RE cells due to opsonisation with immunoglobulin and/or C_3.

marrow shows normal or increased numbers of megakaryocytes. Drug-dependent antibodies against platelets may be demonstrated in the sera of some patients.

The immediate treatment is to stop or replace all suspected drugs. Platelet concentrates are given to patients with dangerous bleeding. Recovery usually occurs after a few hours or days depending on the rapidity of elimination of the drug from the body. These patients must avoid the offending drug and those structurally related to it.

Disseminated intravascular coagulation

Thrombocytopenia may result from an increased rate of platelet destruction through consumption of platelets due to their participation in disseminated intravascular coagulation (p. 233). Initiating factors which may encourage this include damage to endothelium to which the platelets adhere, generalised thrombin formation, viruses, bacteria and endotoxin—all of which produce platelet aggregation. After aggregation, the platelets become trapped in arterioles and capillaries and their level in the circulation falls. One cause of disseminated intravascular platelet aggregation is a disorder known as thrombotic thrombocytopenic purpura (TTP). This condition is characterised by purpura and ischaemic organ damage, e.g. of the brain and kidney.

Increased splenic pooling

Kinetic studies using ⁵¹Cr-labelled platelets indicate that the major factor responsible for thrombocytopenia in splenomegaly is platelet 'pooling' by the spleen. Normally platelets in the general circulation exchange freely with a 'reservoir' or 'pool' of platelets in the splenic microcirculation which accounts for about a third of the total platelet mass. In splenomegaly, the fraction in the exchangeable splenic pool increases and may represent the bulk, e.g. 90% of the marrow output (Fig. 12.5). The platelet lifespan is

Platelet distribution: normal

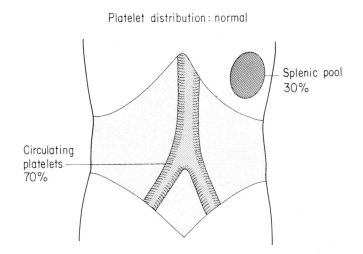

Platelet distribution: splenomegaly

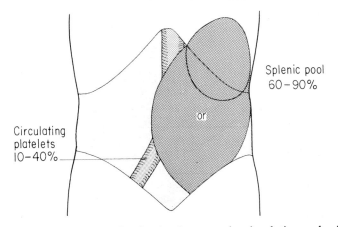

Fig. 12.5 The platelet distribution between the circulation and spleen in normal individuals (*above*) and in patients with moderate or massive splenomegaly (*below*).

Bleeding disorders due to vascular and platelet abnormalities 219

normal since platelets, unlike red cells, tolerate splenic stasis without injury. In the absence of additional haemostatic defects, the thrombocytopenia of splenomegaly is not usually associated with bleeding.

Massive transfusion syndrome

Platelets are unstable in blood stored at 4°C and the platelet count rapidly falls in blood that has been stored for more than 24 hours. Some clotting factors, e.g. factor VIII, also lose activity on storage.

Patients transfused with massive amounts of stored blood (more than 10 units over a 24-hour period) frequently show abnormal bleeding. The defect produced by transfusion with large volumes of stored blood can be minimised if 2 units of fresh blood or blood which is less than 12 hours old is included in every 10 units of blood that is rapidly transfused. Alternatively, platelet concentrates and fresh frozen plasma are used. Established bleeding is treated by administration of fresh whole blood, supplemented if necessary by platelet transfusions and fresh frozen plasma.

DISORDERS OF PLATELET FUNCTION

Disorders of platelet function are suspected in patients who show skin and mucosal haemorrhage and in whom the bleeding time is prolonged despite a normal platelet count. These disorders may be hereditary or acquired.

Hereditary disorders

Rare inherited disorders may produce defects at each of the different phases of the platelet reactions leading to the formation of the haemostatic platelet plug.

In a number of platelet storage pool diseases there is defective release of ADP and 5-hydroxytryptamine due to an intrinsic deficiency in the number of dense granules or α granules.

In thrombasthenia (Glanzmann's disease) there is a failure of primary platelet aggregation. *In the Bernard-Soulier syndrome* the platelets are larger than normal, have a deficiency of a surface glycoprotein, and fail to make phospholipid available or to adhere to vessel walls.

In von Willebrand's disease there is defective platelet adhesion as well as coagulation factor VIII deficiency (see p. 230).

Other rare defects include failure of thromboxane synthesis due to cyclo-oxygenase deficiency and defects of response to thromboxane.

Acquired disorders

Aspirin therapy produces an abnormal bleeding time and, although purpura is unusual, the defect may contribute to the associated gastrointestinal haemorrhage. The cause of the aspirin defect is inhibition of prostaglandin synthetase with impaired thromboxane A_2 synthesis (Fig. 11.4). There is failure of the release reaction and aggregation with adrenalin and ADP. After a single dose the defect lasts 4–7 days. A similar inhibition of platelet function occurs with sulphinpyrazone.

Hyperglobulinaemia associated with multiple myeloma or Waldenström's disease may cause interference with platelet adherence, release and aggregation. *Uraemia* and *liver disease* are also associated with variable abnormalities of platelet function.

Myeloproliferative disorders. Intrinsic abnormalities of platelet function occur in many patients with essential thrombocythaemia and other myeloproliferative diseases.

Antiplatelet drugs

Several clinical trials have assessed the antithrombotic effect of drugs which suppress platelet function. The evidence that these drugs are useful in preventing major thromboembolic disease varies with different clinical situations.

Aspirin is widely used in thrombocytosis where it appears to be effective in preventing thrombosis. The evidence for it being of significant value in patients with ischaemic heart disease is not convincing. In men who have had transient ischaemic attacks, however, aspirin has been shown to reduce significantly the incidence of further attacks, major strokes and death. Sulphinpyrazone may reduce the frequency of sudden death in patients who leave hospital after a myocardial infarct. This antiplatelet agent has also been effective in reducing the frequency of blockage in A-V shunts of chronic dialysis patients and recently prostacyclin has been shown also to be effective for this.

Dipyridamole has been shown to reduce thromboembolic complications in patients with prosthetic heart valves and to improve results in coronary artery by-pass operations.

Laboratory diagnosis of platelet disorders

As thrombocytopenia is the commonest cause of abnormal bleeding, patients with suspected platelet or blood vessel abnormalities should initially have a blood count and blood film examination (see Fig. 12.6). In addition to establishing the presence of thrombocytopenia, the cause of this may be obvious, e.g. acute leukaemia. Bone marrow examination is essential in thrombocytopenic patients to determine whether or not there is a failure of

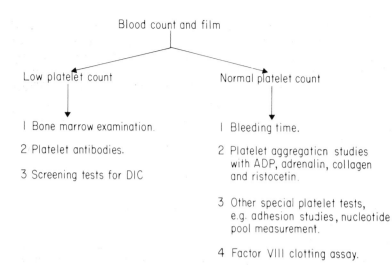

Blood count and film

Low platelet count

↓

1 Bone marrow examination.

2 Platelet antibodies.

3 Screening tests for DIC

Normal platelet count

↓

1 Bleeding time.

2 Platelet aggregation studies with ADP, adrenalin, collagen and ristocetin.

3 Other special platelet tests, e.g. adhesion studies, nucleotide pool measurement.

4 Factor VIII clotting assay.

Fig. 12.6 Laboratory tests for platelet disorders.

platelet production and one of the conditions associated with this (see Table 12.1). In patients with a negative drug history, normal or excessive numbers of marrow megakaryocytes and no other marrow abnormality, ITP is the usual diagnosis. Tests for platelet antibodies or screening tests for disseminated intravascular coagulation may confirm which of the causes of consumptive thrombocytopenia is responsible for the thrombocytopenia.

When the blood count, platelet count and film examination are all normal the bleeding time is done to detect abnormal platelet function. This test measures platelet plug formation *in vivo*. Bleeding stops normally in 3–8 minutes.

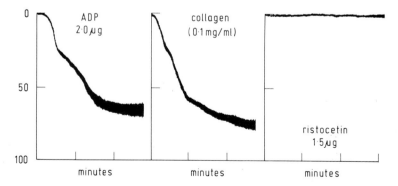

Fig. 12.7 Platelet aggregation with ADP, collagen and ristocetin in von Willebrand's disease. Aggregation is measured by increase in light transmission through a suspension of platelets. Ordinate shows percentage light transmission.

In most patients with abnormal platelet function demonstrated by prolonged bleeding time, the defect is acquired and associated either with systemic disease (e.g. uraemia) or with aspirin therapy. The very rare hereditary defects of platelet function require more elaborate *in vitro* tests to define the specific abnormality. These include platelet aggregation studies with ADP, adrenalin, collagen and ristocetin (Fig. 12.7). If von Willebrand's disease is suspected, factor VIII assays are required.

SELECTED BIBLIOGRAPHY

Belluci S. *et al* (1983) Inherited platelet disorders. *Progress in Hematology*, *XIII*, 223–64. Ed. E.B. Brown. Grune and Stratton, New York.

British Medical Bulletin (1977) **33**, no. 3, *Haemostasis*. Ed. D.P. Thomas.

British Medical Bulletin (1978) **34**, no. 2, *Thrombosis*. Ed. D.P. Thomas.

Clinics in Haematology (1983) vol. 12.1, *Platelet Disorders*. Eds. L.A. Harker & T.S. Zimmerman. W.B. Saunders, Philadelphia.

Weiss H.J. (1975) Platelet physiology and abnormalities of platelet function. *New Engl. J. Med.* **293**, 531.

Weiss H.J. (1978) Antiplatelet therapy. *New Engl. J. Med.* **298**, 1344.

Major references on haemostasis (see Chapter 11).

Major textbooks of haematology (see Chapter 1).

Chapter 13
Coagulation disorders

Hereditary deficiencies of each of ten coagulation factors have been described. Haemophilia A (factor VIII deficiency), haemophilia B (Christmas disease, factor IX deficiency) and von Willebrand's disease are uncommon; the others are rare.

HAEMOPHILIA A

Haemophilia is the most common hereditary disorder of blood coagulation. The inheritance is sex-linked (Fig. 13.1) but 33% of

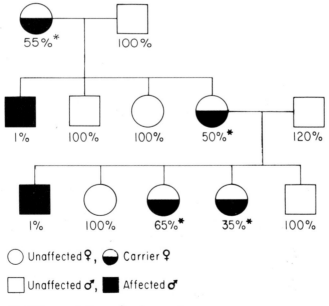

○ Unaffected ♀, ◐ Carrier ♀

☐ Unaffected ♂, ■ Affected ♂

%=$\underline{VIII}$: c activity as % of normal

Fig. 13.1 A typical family tree in a family with haemophilia. Note variable levels of factor VIII activity in carriers (*) due to random inactivation of X chromosome (Lyonisation).

patients have no family history and presumably result from recent spontaneous mutation. The incidence is of the order of 1 per 10 000 population.

The defect is an absence or low level of plasma factor VIII clotting activity (VIII:C). It appears likely that there is either defective synthesis of this part of factor VIII or synthesis of a structurally abnormal molecule. Immunological studies show normal amounts of factor VIII-related antigen (VIIIR:AG). The factor VIII component concerned with the platelet adhesion mediating function of VIIIR:AG (VIII:VWF) is also unaffected (Fig. 13.2).

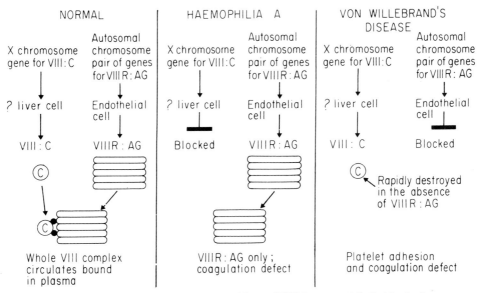

Fig. 13.2 The synthesis of factor VIII in normal individuals, in haemophilia A and in von Willebrand's disease.

Clinical features

Severely affected infants may suffer from profuse post-circumcision haemorrhage. Recurrent painful haemarthroses and muscle haematomas dominate the clinical course—with progressive deformity and crippling (Figs. 13.3a, b & c). Prolonged bleeding occurs after dental extractions. Haematuria is more common than gastrointestinal haemorrhage. Operative and post-traumatic haemorrhage are life-threatening both in severely and mildly affected patients. Although not common, spontaneous intracerebral haemorrhage occurs more frequently than in the general population and is an important cause of death in patients with severe disease.

The clinical severity of the disease correlates well with extent of the coagulation factor deficiency (Table 13.1).

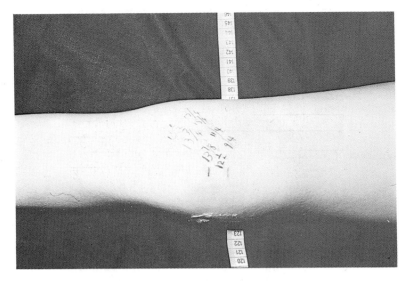

Fig. 13.3a An acute haemarthrosis of the knee joint in a patient with haemophilia. The changes in circumference of the joint with treatment are indicated.

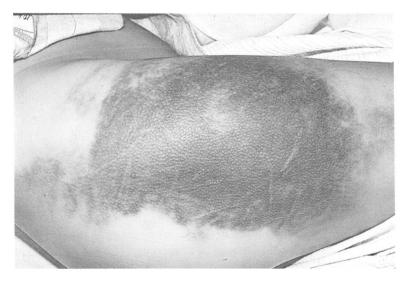

Fig. 13.3b A massive haematoma of the buttock in a patient with haemophilia.

It is becoming apparent that many haemophiliacs have subclinical liver disease, and a few show clinical features of chronic hepatitis. It is likely that this is largely due to the many infusions of blood products and consequent exposure to hepatitis B, or non-A, non-B hepatitis virus. AIDS has been described in rare cases.

Haemophilic pseudotumours may occur in the long bones,

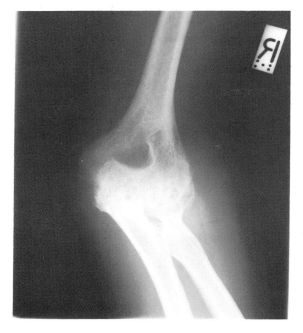

Fig. 13.3c Radiographic appearances of the right elbow joint in a 25-year-old male with haemophilia. The joint space has been destroyed and there is bony ankylosis. Subchondral cystic areas are prominent.

Table 13.1 Correlation of coagulation factor activity and disease severity in haemophilia and factor IX deficiency.

Coagulation factor activity (% of normal)	Clinical manifestations
< 1	Severe disease. Frequent spontaneous bleeding episodes from early life. Joint deformity and crippling if not adequately treated
1–5	Moderate disease. Post-traumatic bleeding. Occasional spontaneous episodes
5–20	Mild disease. Post-traumatic bleeding

pelvis, fingers and toes. These result from repeated sub-periosteal haemorrhages with bone destruction, new bone formation, expansion of the bone and pathological fractures.

Drug addiction due to repeated need for analgesics is a problem in some teenagers or adults with severe disease and progressive joint destruction.

Laboratory diagnosis (see Table 13.2)

The following tests are abnormal:
(i) Activated partial thromboplastin time (APTT or PTTK).
(ii) Whole blood coagulation time (severe cases).
(iii) Factor VIII clotting assay (VIII:C).
Immunological methods show normal VIIIR:AG. The bleeding time and prothrombin time tests are also normal.

Carrier females may be identified with reasonable confidence since they show only half the VIII:C activity expected for the level of VIIIR:AG. Antenatal diagnosis and abortion of affected foetuses is now possible since low levels of VIII:C have been demonstrated in blood samples obtained by direct vision foetoscopy from affected foetuses.

Table 13.2 Main clinical and laboratory findings in haemophilia A, factor IX deficiency (haemophilia B, Christmas disease) and von Willebrand's diease.

	Haemophilia A	Factor IX deficiency	Von Willebrand's disease
Inheritance	Sex-linked	⎫	Dominant (incomplete)
Main sites of haemorrhage	Muscle, joints post-trauma or operation	⎬ as haemophilia A ⎭	Mucous membranes, skin cuts, post-trauma and operation
Platelet count	Normal	Normal	Normal
Bleeding time	Normal	Normal	Prolonged
Prothrombin time	Normal	Normal	Normal
Partial thromboplastin time	Prolonged	Prolonged	Prolonged or normal
Factor VIII:C	Low	Normal	Low
Factor VIII:AG	Normal	Normal	Low
Factor IX	Normal	Low	Normal
Ristocetin-induced platelet aggregation	Normal	Normal	Impaired

CKT

Treatment

Bleeding episodes are treated with factor VIII replacement therapy or by the administration of desmopressin (DDAVP). Factor VIII levels are raised most effectively with infusions of plasma cryoprecipitate or factor VIII concentrates. Spontaneous bleeding is controlled if the patient's factor VIII level is raised above 20% of normal. For major surgery, serious post-traumatic bleeding or when haemorrhage is occurring at a dangerous site, however, the factor VIII level should be elevated to 100% and then maintained above 60% when acute bleeding has stopped, until healing has occurred.

Desmopressin provides an alternative means of increasing the plasma factor VIII level, particularly in milder haemophiliacs. Following the intravenous administration of this drug there is a moderate rise in the patient's own factor VIII which is proportional to the resting level. Desmopressin may also be inhaled as snuff— this is particularly useful as immediate treatment for mild haemophiliacs after accidental trauma or haemorrhage.

Local supportive measures used in treating haemarthroses and haematomas include resting the affected part and the prevention of further trauma.

The increased availability of factor VIII concentrates which may be stored in domestic refrigerators has dramatically altered haemophilia treatment. At the earliest suggestion of bleeding the haemophiliac child may be treated at home. This advance has reduced the occurrence of crippling haemarthroses and the need for in-patient care.

Haemophiliacs are advised to have regular conservative dental care. Haemophiliac children and their parents often require extensive help with social and psychological matters. With modern treatment the life-style of a haemophilic child can be almost normal but certain activities such as body contact sports are to be avoided.

One of the most serious complications of haemophilia is the development of antibodies (inhibitors) to isologous factor VIII which occurs in 5–10% of patients. This renders the patient refractory to further replacement therapy so that tremendous doses have to be given to achieve a significant rise in plasma factor VIII:C activity. Immunosuppression has been used in an attempt to reduce formation of the antibody. Some factor IX concentrates contain activated factor X. A special preparation known as FEIBA (factor eight inhibitor bypassing activity) has been used successfully in the treatment of severe haemorrhage in these patients. Porcine factor VIII concentrates have also been effective in some patients.

FACTOR IX DEFICIENCY

The inheritance and clinical features of factor IX deficiency (Christmas disease, haemophilia B) are identical to those of haemophilia A. Indeed the two disorders can only be distinguished by specific coagulation factor assays. The incidence is one-fifth that of haemophilia A. Many patients have immunochemical evidence for the presence of a functionally defective factor IX protein.

Laboratory diagnosis (see Table 13.2)

The following tests are abnormal:
(i) Activated partial thromboplastin time.
(ii) Whole blood clotting time (severe cases).
(iii) Factor IX clotting assay.

As in haemophilia A the bleeding time and prothrombin time tests are normal.

Treatment

The principles of replacement therapy are similar to those of hae-mophilia. Bleeding episodes are treated with factor IX concen-trates. Because of the stability *in vitro* of factor IX, stored plasma is also effective. Because of its longer biological half-life, infusions do not have to be given as frequently as factor VIII concentrates in haemophilia.

VON WILLEBRAND'S DISEASE

In this disorder abnormal platelet adhesion is associated with low factor VIII clotting activity. The introduction of more reliable tests for this condition and the awareness that clinical features may be mild has changed the previous concept that the condition is rare. The true incidence may be similar to, or even exceed, that of haemophilia. The inheritance is autosomal dominant with vary-ing expression. The primary defect appears to be a reduced syn-thesis of the major fraction of factor VIII, VIIIR:AG. The plate-let-related activities of factor VIII (von Willebrand factor) such as the potentiation of platelet adherence to subendothelial con-nective tissue or glass and its participation in ristocetin-induced platelet aggregation are probably the result of a particular molecular configuration of the VIIIR:AG molecule (Fig. 11.3).

The bleeding is characterised by operative and post-traumatic haemorrhage, mucous membrane bleeding (e.g. epistaxes, men-orrhagia) and excessive blood loss from superficial cuts and abrasions. Haemarthroses and muscle haematomas are rare, except in homozygous cases.

Laboratory diagnosis (see Table 13.2)

(i) Prolonged bleeding time.
(ii) Low levels of factor VIII clotting activity (VIII:C).
(iii) Low levels of VIII-related antigen (VIIIR:AG).
(iv) Defective platelet aggregation with ristocetin. Ristocetin, an antibiotic which was withdrawn because of its side-effect of

thrombocytopenia, induces platelet aggregation in normal plate-let-rich plasma, but not in patients with von Willebrand's disease. The aggregation response to other agents (ADP, collagen, thrombin, adrenalin) is normal (Fig. 12.7).

(v) Low VIII:VWF activity in patient's plasma (assay uses ristocetin-treated donor 'pool' platelets).

(vi) In some patients there is defective retention of platelets in glass bead columns.

The laboratory results in mildly affected patients are somewhat variable.

Treatment

Bleeding episodes are treated with cryoprecipitate, factor VIII concentrates or desmopressin. Factor VIII infusions may be associated with sustained and often delayed increases of factor VIII clotting activity (Fig. 13.4).

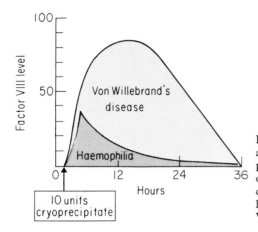

Fig. 13.4 Comparison of activity of factor VIII:C in plasma following infusion of factor VIII (as cryoprecipitate) in haemophilia and von Willebrand's disease.

HEREDITARY DISORDERS OF OTHER COAGULATION FACTORS

All these disorders are rare. In most the inheritance is autosomal. There is usually a good correlation between the patient's symptoms and the severity of the coagulation deficiency; however, there are exceptions. Factor XII deficiency is not associated with abnormal bleeding and, although factor XI deficiency produces a marked laboratory defect, the clinical symptoms are mild. Factor XIII deficiency produces a severe bleeding tendency but the usual screening tests for coagulation disorders are normal. A test of clot stability in the presence of 5 M urea is required to reveal this rare autosomal recessive defect.

Acquired VITAMIN K DEFICIENCY

Fat soluble vitamin K is obtained from green vegetables and bacterial synthesis in the gut. Deficiency may present in the newborn (haemorrhagic disease of the newborn) or in later life.

Haemorrhagic disease of the newborn

Vitamin K-dependent factors are low at birth and fall further in breast-fed infants in the first few days of life. Liver cell immaturity, lack of gut bacterial synthesis of the vitamin and low quantities in breast milk may all contribute to deficiency which may cause haemorrhage usually on the 2nd–4th day of life.

DIAGNOSIS. The prothrombin time (PT) and activated partial thromboplastin time (APTT) are both abnormal. The platelet counts and fibrinogen are normal with absent fibrin degradation products.

TREATMENT
(i) Prophylaxis: vitamin K (Konakion) 1 mg intramuscularly after birth is given to all new-born babies.
(ii) In bleeding infants: vitamin K 1 mg i.m. is given every six hours with, initially, fresh frozen plasma if haemorrhage is severe.
   A good response is usual in healthy full-term babies. Because of liver cell immaturity the response in premature babies is often suboptimal. If bleeding is not controlled with vitamin K, fresh blood or plasma may be necessary.

Vitamin K deficiency in children or adults

Deficiency resulting from obstructive jaundice, pancreatic or small bowel disease occasionally causes a bleeding diathesis in children or adults.

DIAGNOSIS. Both the prothrombin time and APTT (or PTTK) are prolonged. There are low levels of factor II, VII, IX and X in plasma.

TREATMENT
(i) Prophylaxis: vitamin K 5 mg orally each day.
(ii) Active bleeding or prior to liver biopsy: vitamin K 10 mg subcutaneously. Some correction of prothrombin time is usual within six hours. The dose should be repeated on the next two days after which time optimal correction is usual.

LIVER DISEASE

Multiple haemostatic abnormalities contribute to a bleeding tendency and may exacerbate haemorrhage from oesophageal varices.

(i) Biliary obstruction results in impaired absorption of vitamin K and therefore decreased synthesis of factor II, VII, IX and X by liver parenchymal cells.
(ii) With severe hepatocellular disease, in addition to a deficiency of these factors there are often reduced levels of factor V and fibrinogen and increased amounts of plasminogen activator.
(iii) Hypersplenism associated with portal hypertension frequently results in thrombocytopenia.
(iv) Patients in liver failure have variable platelet functional abnormalities.
(v) Functional abnormality of fibrinogen (dysfibrinogenaemia) is found in many patients.

DISSEMINATED INTRAVASCULAR COAGULATION (DIC)

Widespread intravascular deposition of fibrin with consumption of coagulation factors and platelets occurs as a consequence of many disorders which release procoagulant material into the circulation or cause widespread endothelial damage or platelet aggregation. It may be associated with a fulminant haemorrhagic syndrome or run a less severe and more chronic course.

Pathogenesis

1 DIC may be triggered by entry of procoagulant material into the circulation in the following situations: amniotic fluid embolism, premature separation of the placenta, widespread mucin-secreting adenocarcinoma, promyelocytic leukaemia, severe falciparum malaria, haemolytic transfusion reaction, and some snake bites.
2 DIC may also be initiated by widespread endothelial damage and collagen exposure, for example endotoxaemia, Gram-negative and meningococcal septicaemia, septic abortion; certain virus infections (e.g. purpura fulminans); and severe burns or hypothermia.
3 Widespread intravascular platelet aggregation may also precipitate DIC. Some bacteria, viruses and immune complexes may have a direct effect on platelets.

In addition to its role in the deposition of fibrin in the microcirculation, intravascular thrombin formation produces large amounts of circulating fibrin monomers which form complexes with available fibrinogen. Intense fibrinolysis is stimulated by thrombi on vascular walls and the release of split products interferes with fibrin polymerisation, thus contributing to the coagulation defect. The combined action of thrombin and plasmin normally causes depletion of fibrinogen, prothrombin, factor V and factor VIII. Intravascular thrombin also causes widespread platelet aggregation, release and deposition. The bleeding problems of DIC are compounded by the inevitable thrombocytopenia due to consumption of platelets.

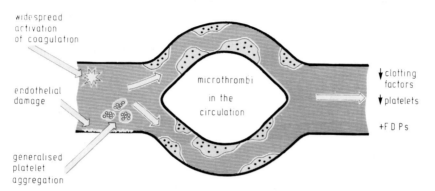

Fig. 13.5 The pathogenesis of disseminated intravascular coagulation and the changes in clotting factors, platelets and fibrin degradation products (FDPs) that occur in this syndrome.

Laboratory diagnosis

In many acute syndromes the blood may fail to clot because of gross fibrinogen deficiency.

TESTS OF HAEMOSTASIS
(i) The platelet count is low.
(ii) Fibrinogen screening tests, titres or assays indicate deficiency.
(iii) The thrombin time is prolonged.
(iv) Tests for fibrin monomer complex (e.g. ethanol gelation test) are positive.
(v) High levels of fibrinogen (and fibrin) degradation products are found in serum and urine.
(vi) PT and APTT are prolonged in the acute syndromes.
(vii) Factor V and factor VIII activities are reduced.
In more chronic syndromes increased synthesis of coagulation factors may result in normal assays and screening test results. Tests for systemic fibrinolysis (euglobulin clot lysis) usually show no increase in circulating plasminogen activator.

BLOOD FILM EXAMINATION. In many patients there is a haemolytic anaemia ('microangiopathic') and the red cells show
prominent fragmentation due to damage passing through fibrin
strands in small vessels (see p. 83).

Treatment of DIC

(i) Treatment of the underlying causative disorder is most important.
(ii) Supportive therapy with fresh blood, fresh frozen plasma,
fibrinogen and platelet concentrates is indicated in patients with
dangerous or extensive bleeding.
(iii) The use of heparin or antiplatelet drugs to inhibit the coagulation process is controversial since bleeding may, in some cases,
be aggravated.

COAGULATION DEFICIENCY CAUSED BY ANTIBODIES

Circulating antibodies to coagulation factors are occasionally seen.
Allo-antibodies to factor VIII occur in 5–10% of haemophiliacs.
Factor VIII auto-antibodies may also result in a bleeding
syndrome. These IgG antibodies occur rarely *post-partum*, in certain immunological disorders (e.g. rheumatoid arthritis), and in old
age. Many of these antibodies combine with and inactivate the
coagulation protein but do not lead to premature removal of the
protein from the circulation.

ANTICOAGULANT DRUGS

Anticoagulant drugs are used widely in the treatment of venous
thromboembolic disease. Their value in the treatment of arterial
thrombosis is less well established. Heparin and the oral anticoagulants are considered here.

Heparin

This acidic mucopolysaccharide is a direct inhibitor of blood
coagulation. As it is not absorbed from the gastrointestinal tract,
it must be given by injection. It is inactivated by the liver and
excreted in the urine. The effective biological half-life is about one
hour.

MODE OF ACTION. Heparin dramatically potentiates the formation of complexes between antithrombin III and activated serine

protease coagulation factors which are thrombin, factors XIIa, XIa, Xa, IXa and VIIa (Fig. 13.6). This complex formation inactivates these factors irreversibly.

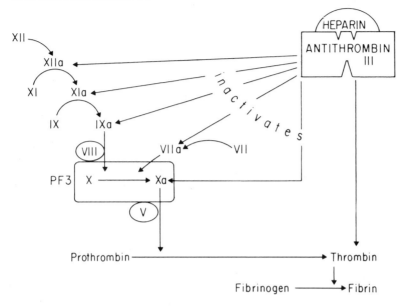

Fig. 13.6 The action of heparin. This activates antithrombin III which then forms complexes with activated serine protease coagulation factors (XIIa, XIa, Xa, IXa, VIIa and thrombin) and so inactivates them.

ADMINISTRATION AND LABORATORY CONTROL

1 *Continuous intravenous infusion* provides the smoothest control of heparin therapy and is the recommended method of administration. In an adult, doses of 30–40 000 units over 24 hours are usually satisfactory. Therapy is monitored by maintaining the whole blood coagulation time at twice normal, or the activated partial thromboplastin time (which is a more accurate test) at between $1\frac{1}{2}$ and 2 times the normal time.

2 *Intermittent subcutaneous injections* are preferred when heparin is given as prophylaxis against venous thrombosis. This method is also useful when long-term treatment is indicated. The usual dose is 5000–10 000 units 12 hourly. Long-term treatment may have the serious side-effect of osteoporosis due to complexing mineral substance from bone.

BLEEDING DURING HEPARIN THERAPY. Intravenous heparin has a half-life of less than one hour and it is usually only necessary to stop the infusion. Protamine is able to inactivate heparin immediately and for severe bleeding a dose of 1 mg/100 units of heparin provides effective neutralisation. However, protamine itself may act as an anticoagulant.

Oral anticoagulants

The oral anticoagulants are derivatives of coumarin or indanedione. Warfarin, a coumarin derivative, is most widely used. It is well absorbed from the gut, and it is usual to start treatment with 5–10 mg and alter the dose according to the results of the prothrombin time.

MODE OF ACTION. These drugs are vitamin K antagonists. Therapy results in decreased biological activity of the vitamin K-dependent factors II, VII, IX and X. Oral anticoagulants block the post ribosomal γ carboxylation of glutamic acid residues of these proteins (Fig. 11.7) and the resulting abnormal molecules—known as 'proteins induced by vitamin K absence or antagonism' (PIVKA)—are released into the cirulation (Fig. 13.7). After warfarin is given, factor VII levels fall considerably within 24 hours

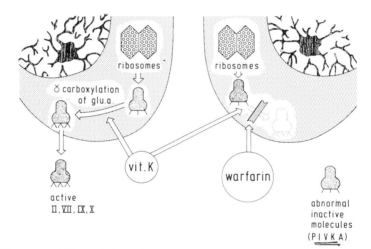

Fig. 13.7 The action of vitamin K in γ carboxylation of factors II (prothrombin), VII, IX and X. Oral anticoagulants (e.g. warfarin) are vitamin K antagonists and lead to accumulation in plasma of inactive molecules (PIVKA).

but prothrombin has longer plasma half-life and only falls to 50% of normal at 3 days, and the patient is fully anticoagulated only after this period.

LABORATORY CONTROL. The effect of oral anticoagulants may be monitored by either prothrombin time (using plasma) or thrombotest (using whole blood). Therapy is adjusted to keep the prothrombin time between two and four times that of the control (Fig. 13.8), or the thrombotest between 5 and 15%.

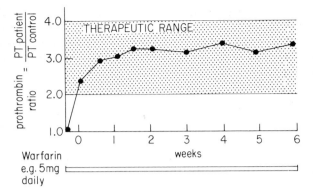

Fig. 13.8 The laboratory control of oral anticoagulant therapy using the prothrombin ratio.

DRUG INTERACTION. About 97% of warfarin in the circulation is albumin-bound and it is the small fraction of warfarin that is free and can enter the liver parenchymal cell which is active. In the liver cell, warfarin is degraded in microsomes to an inactive water soluble metabolite which is conjugated and excreted in the bile

Table 13.3 Factors interfering with the control of oral anticoagulant therapy.

Potentiating factors	Inhibiting factors
Drugs which displace anticoagulant from albumin binding in plasma, e.g. aspirin, phenylbutazone, sulphinpyrazone (these also have an antiplatelet action), chlorpromazine. Inhibition of microsomal degradation of anticoagulant, e.g. alcohol, nortryptiline. ↓ synthesis of II, VII, IX, X, e.g. liver disease, phenytoin, salicylates. ↓ absorption of vitamin K, e.g. malabsorption, antibiotics, laxatives.	Drugs which induce microsomal degradation of anticoagulant, e.g. barbiturates, dichloralphenazone, glutethimide. Hereditary resistance to oral anticoagulants. Malignant disease. Oral contraceptives, pregnancy, thiazide diuretics.

and partially re-absorbed to be also excreted in urine. Drugs which affect the albumin binding or excretion of warfarin (or of other oral anticoagulants) interfere with the control of therapy (Table 13.3).

BLEEDING DURING WARFARIN THERAPY. Mild bleeding usually only needs a prothrombin ratio or thrombotest assessment and dosage adjustment. More serious bleeding may need cessation of therapy and the infusion of fresh frozen plasma. Factor concentrates carry the risks of DIC and hepatitis and their use should be restricted to patients who are unable to tolerate the volume of FFP required (1–2 litres). Vitamin $K_1$is the specific antidote: an intravenous injection of 2.5 mg is effective but will result in resistance to further warfarin therapy for 2–3 weeks.

STREPTOKINASE, UROKINASE

These enzymes which activate plasmin have been used to increase fibrinolytic activity of plasma in an attempt to dissolve thrombi. Careful control is needed to avoid serious haemorrhage as a complication.

SELECTED BIBLIOGRAPHY

British Medical Bulletin (1977) **33,** no. 3, *Haemostasis.* Ed. D.P. Thomas.
British Medical Bulletin (1978) **34,** no. 2, *Thrombosis,* Ed. D.P. Thomas.
Clinics in Haematology (1979) vol. 8.1, *Congenital Coagulation Disorders.* Ed. C.R. Rizza. W.B. Saunders, Philadelphia.
Clinics in Haematology (1981) vol. 10.2, *Thrombosis.* Ed. C.R.M. Prentice. W.B. Saunders, Philadelphia.
Ingram G.I.C., Brozovic M. & Slater M.G.P. (1983) *Bleeding Disorders—Investigation and Management,* 2nd edition. Blackwell Scientific Publications, Oxford.
Methods in Haematology (1982) *The Hemophilias.* Ed. A.L. Bloom. Churchill Livingstone, Edinburgh.
Poller L. (ed.) (1977 & 1981) *Recent Advances in Blood Coagulation,* 2nd & 3rd editions. Churchill Livingstone, Edinburgh.
Seminars in Hematology (1977) vols. 14.4. (1978) 15.1; 15.2, *Hemostasis and Thrombosis.* Ed. R.S. Mibasham. Grune and Stratton, New York.
Major references on haemostasis (see Chapter 11).
Major textbooks of haematology (see Chapter 1).

Chapter 14
Blood transfusion

Blood transfusion involves the infusion of whole blood or a blood component from one individual (the donor) to another (the recipient). The major clinical aspect is the transfusion of red cells. Compatibility between donor red cell antigens and the recipient's plasma antibodies must be ensured, otherwise potentially fatal haemolytic reactions may occur. Recent changes in the use of specific blood components has also placed heavy emphasis on platelets, haemostatic agents, plasma protein colloids and immunoglobulins.

Red cell antigens

Approximately 400 blood group antigens have been described. These are inherited in a simple Mendelian fashion and are stable characteristics which are therefore useful in paternity testing. The significance of blood groups in blood transfusions is that individuals who lack a particular blood group antigen may produce antibodies reacting with that antigen. These may lead to a transfusion reaction if red cells bearing the antigen are transfused. Different blood group antigens have different antigenic strength (i.e. antigenicity, or potential for immunising). The ABO and rhesus groups are of major clinical significance. Some other systems of less overall importance are listed in Table 14.1.

Table 14.1 Main blood group systems.

System	Frequency of antibodies	Cause of haemolytic disease of newborn
ABO	Very common (see text)	Yes
Rhesus	Common	Yes
Kell	Occasional	Yes
Duffy	Occasional	Yes
Kidd	Occasional	Yes
Lutheran	Rare	Yes
Lewis	Rare	No
P	Rare	No
MNSs	Rare	No
Ii	Rare	No

Blood group antibodies

Naturally occurring antibodies occur in the serum of subjects who lack the corresponding antigen and who have not been transfused. The most important are anti-A and anti-B. They are usually IgM, and react optimally at cold temperatures (4°C) and are called cold antibodies.

Immune antibodies develop in response to the introduction—by transfusion or by transplacental passage during pregnancy—of red cells possessing antigens which the subject lacks. These antibodies are commonly IgG although some IgM antibodies may also develop—usually in the early phase of an immune response. Immune antibodies react optimally at 37°C (warm antibodies). Only IgG antibodies are capable of transplacental passage from mother to foetus. An important immune antibody is the rhesus antibody, anti-D.

ABO SYSTEM

This consists of three allelic genes: A, B and O. The A and B genes control the synthesis of specific enzymes responsible for the addition of single carbohydrate residues (N-acetylgalactosamine for Group A and D-galactose for Group B) to a basic antigenic glycoprotein with a terminal sugar L-fucose on the red cell, known as the H substance. The O gene is an amorph and does not transform the H substance. Although there are six possible genotypes, the absence of a specific anti-O prevents the recognition of more than four phenotypes (see Table 14.2). Sub-groups of A complicate the issue but are of minor clinical significance. A_1 and A_2 are commonly distinguished. A_2 cells react more weakly with anti-A than A_1 cells and patients who are A_2B can be wrongly grouped as B.

The A, B and H antigens are present on most body cells including white cells and platelets. In the 80% of the population who possess secretor genes, these antigens are also found in soluble form in tissues and body fluids, e.g. plasma, saliva, semen and

Table 14.2 ABO blood group system.

Phenotype	Genotype	Antigens	Naturally-occurring antibodies	Frequency (U.K.) %
O	*OO*	O	Anti-A, B	46
A	*AA* or *AO*	A	Anti-B	42
B	*BB* or *BO*	B	Anti-A	9
AB	*AB*	AB	None	3

sweat. The stability of ABO antigens allows their detection on dried blood stains and semen and this is important in forensic medicine.

Naturally-occurring antibodies to A and/or B antigen are found in the plasma of subjects whose red cells lack the corresponding antigens (Table 14.2).

RHESUS SYSTEM

This complex system is coded by allelic genes at three closely linked loci; alternative antigens Cc, Ee together with D or no D (termed 'd') exist. Thus a person may inherit CDe from the mother and cde from the father to have a genotype CDe/cde. There is a shortened nomenclature for these linked sets of genes — the 'R' nomenclature shown in Table 14.3.

Table 14.3 Rhesus system — genotypes.

CDE nomenclature	Short symbol	Caucasian frequency (%)	Rhesus D status
cde/cde	rr	15	Negative
CDe/cde	R_1r	32	Positive
CDe/CDe	R_1R_1	17	Positive
cDE/cde	R_2r	13	Positive
CDe/cDE	R_1R_2	14	Positive
cDE/cDE	R_2R_2	4	Positive
Other genotypes		5	Positive (almost all)

Rhesus antibodies are *immune*, since they result from previous transfusion or pregnancy. Anti-D is responsible for most of the clinical problems associated with the system and a simple subdivision of subjects into rhesus D positive and rhesus D negative using anti-D is sufficient for routine clinical purposes. Anti-C, anti-c, anti-E and anti-e are occasionally seen and may cause both transfusion reactions and haemolytic disease of the newborn. Anti-d is thought not to exist. Rhesus haemolytic disease of the newborn is described later in this chapter.

OTHER BLOOD GROUP SYSTEMS

Other blood group systems are less frequently of clinical importance. Although naturally-occurring antibodies of the P, Lewis and MN system are not uncommon they usually only react at low temperatures. Immune antibodies against antigens of these systems are detected infrequently. Many of the antigens are of low antigenicity and others (e.g. Kell), although comparatively anti-genic, are of relatively low frequency and therefore provide few opportunities for iso-immunisation.

TECHNIQUES IN BLOOD GROUP SEROLOGY

The following techniques are used. They rely on the identification visually or microscopically of the agglutination of red cells.

1. *Saline agglutination.* This is important in detecting cold anti-bodies (mainly IgM) at room temperature and 4°C. Antibodies are often described as saline, or complete agglutinins.

2. *Addition of colloid.* Albumin, polyvinylpyrroldone.

3. *Enzyme treatment of red cells,* e.g. papain, bromelin, ficin.

4. *Low ionic strength saline (LISS).*

The use of colloids, enzymes or LISS modify either the media in which the red cells are suspended or the red cell surface, and permit the cells to come closer together. This facilitates agglutination by many IgG (or IgA) antibodies, which cannot produce agglutination in a saline suspension of red cells.

In the case of rhesus-D, an international standard of antibody has been prepared and it is possible to quantitate the amount of antibody present in a serum. This is of some clinical value in managing pregnant women in cases of haemolytic disease of the newborn (see later).

5. *The Coombs' test,* see below.

The Coombs' test

This is a fundamental and widely used test in both blood group serology and general immunology. Anti-human globulin (AHG) may be produced in various animals (e.g. rabbits and horses) fol-lowing the injection of human globulin or purified complement or specific immunoglobulin (e.g. IgG, IgA or IgM). When purified animal AHG is added to human red cells coated with immuno-globulin or complement components, agglutination of the red cells indicates a positive test (Fig. 14.1).

DIRECT COOMBS' TEST

This is used for detecting antibody or complement on the red cell surface where sensitisation has occurred *in vivo*. The AHG re-agent is added to washed red cells and agglutination indicates a positive test.

A positive direct Coombs' test occurs in:

a   haemolytic disease of the newborn,

b   auto-immune haemolytic anaemia,

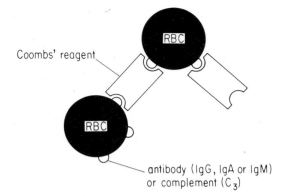

Fig. 14.1 The Coombs' test for antibody or complement on the surface of red cells. The Coombs' (anti human globulin, AHG) reagent may be broad spectrum or specific for IgG, IgM, IgA or complement (C_3).

Coombs' reagent

RBC

RBC

antibody (IgG, IgA or IgM) or complement (C_3)

c drug-induced immune haemolytic anaemia,
d haemolytic transfusion reactions.

INDIRECT COOMBS' TEST

This is used to detect blood group antibodies in serum. It is a two-stage procedure: the first step involves the incubation of test red cells with serum; in the second step, the red cells are thoroughly washed with saline to remove free globulins. The AHG reagent is then added to the washed red cells. Agglutination in the test implies that the original serum contained antibody which has coated the red cells *in vitro*. This test is used:
a as part of the routine cross-matching procedure for the detection of antibodies in the patient against donor red cells;
b for detecting atypical blood group antibodies in serum during screening procedures;
c for detecting blood group antibodies in a pregnant woman;
d for detecting antibodies in serum in auto-immune haemolytic anaemia.

SPECIFICITY OF AHG

A broad spectrum reagent is usually preferred in normal blood transfusion procedures as it detects both antibodies and complement components. Monospecific AHG reagents include anti-IgG, anti-IgM, anti-IgA, anti-C_3, and anti-C_4. These are used in detailed investigations on the nature of blood group antibodies, particularly in haemolytic anaemias.

Cross-matching pre-transfusion tests

Prior to blood transfusion the blood group of the patient is determined, the serum is screened for atypical antibodies, and red cells from each donor unit are tested against the patient's serum (the cross-match, Table 14.4).

Blood of the same ABO and rhesus D group is selected. The cross-match normally takes about one hour. When blood is required urgently, the tests may be carried out quickly by limiting the tests performed and modifying the techniques. This does reduce test sensitivity but will detect all gross incompatibilities. Transfusion of un-cross-matched blood in emergencies carries considerable risk and should be avoided when possible. When the urgency of a clinical situation does not allow time for grouping the patient, group O rhesus negative blood should be transfused.

Table 14.4 Techniques used in compatibility testing.

Donor cells tested against recipient serum and agglutination detected visually or microscopically after mixing and incubation at the appropriate temperature.

For detecting cold antibodies (mainly IgM)
Saline room temperature

For detecting immune antibodies (mainly IgG)
Albumin addition at 37°C
Enzyme-treated red cells at 37°C
Low ionic strength saline at 37°C
Indirect Coombs' test at 37°C

COMPLICATIONS OF BLOOD TRANSFUSION

Haemolytic transfusion reactions

Haemolytic transfusion reactions may be immediate or delayed. Immediate life-threatening reactions associated with massive intravascular haemolysis are the result of complement-activating antibodies of IgM or IgG classes (e.g. ABO antibodies). The severity of the reaction depends on the recipient's titre of antibody; severe reactions are rare with other antibodies. Reactions associated with extravascular haemolysis (e.g. immune antibodies of the rhesus system which are unable to activate complement) are generally less severe but may still be life-threatening. The cells become coated with IgG and are removed in the RE system. In mild cases, the only signs of a transfusion reaction may be a progressive unexplained anaemia with or without jaundice. In some cases where the pre-transfusion level of an antibody was too low to be detected in a cross-match, a patient may be re-immunised by transfusion of incompatible red cells and this will lead to a delayed transfusion reaction with accelerated clearance of the red cells. There may be rapid appearance of anaemia with mild jaundice.

CLINICAL FEATURES OF A MAJOR HAEMOLYTIC
TRANSFUSION REACTION

(i) *Haemolytic shock phase.* This may occur after only a few ml of blood or up to one to two hours after the end of the transfusion.

Table 14.5 Complications of blood transfusion.

Early	Late

Haemolytic reactions
  Immediate
  Delayed
	Transmission of disease e.g.
	  hepatitis, malaria, syphilis,
	  cytomegalovirus, AIDS

Reactions due to infected blood	Transfusional iron overload

Allergic reactions to white cells,
  platelets or proteins
	Immune sensitisation, e.g. to
	  rhesus D antigen

Pyrogenic reactions (to plasma
  proteins or due to HLA
  antibodies)	

Circulatory overload	
Air embolism	
Thrombophlebitis	
Citrate toxicity	
Hyperkalaemia	
Clotting abnormalities (after massive transfusion)	

Clinical features include urticaria, pain in the lumbar region, flushing, headache, precordial pain, shortness of breath, vomiting, rigors, pyrexia and a fall in blood pressure. If the patient is anaesthetised this shock phase is masked. There is increasing evidence of blood destruction and haemoglobinuria, jaundice and disseminated intravascular coagulation may occur. Moderate leucocytosis, e.g. $15–20 \times 10^9/l$ is usual.

(ii) *The oliguric phase.* In some patients with a haemolytic reaction there is renal tubular necrosis with acute renal failure.

(iii) *Diuretic phase.* Fluid and electrolyte imbalance may occur during the recovery from acute renal failure.

INVESTIGATION OF AN IMMEDIATE TRANSFUSION REACTION

If a patient develops features suggesting a severe transfusion reaction, the transfusion should be stopped and investigations for blood group incompatibility and bacterial contamination of the blood must be initiated.

1 Most severe reactions occur because of clerical errors in handling donor or recipient's blood specimens. Therefore it must be established that the identity of the recipient is the same as that stated on the compatibility label and that this corresponds with the actual unit being transfused.

2 The unit of blood and post-transfusion samples of the patient's blood should be sent to the laboratory who will:

   a Repeat the group on pre- and post-transfusion samples and on the blood, and repeat the cross-match.

   b Do a direct Coombs' test on the post-transfusion sample.

c Check the plasma for haemoglobinaemia.

d Perform tests for disseminated intravascular coagulation.

e Examine the donor sample directly for evidence of gross bacterial contamination and set up blood cultures from it at 20°C and 37°C.

3 A post-transfusion sample of urine must be examined for haemoglobinuria.

4 Further samples of blood are taken at 6 and/or 24 hours after transfusion for blood counting and bilirubin, free haemoglobin and methaemalbumin estimations.

5 In the absence of positive findings, the patient's serum is examined 5–10 days later for red cell or white cell antibodies.

MANAGEMENT OF PATIENTS WITH MAJOR HAEMOLYSIS

The principal object of initial therapy is to maintain the blood pressure and renal perfusion. Intravenous dextran, plasma or saline and frusemide are usually given. Hydrocortisone 100 mg i.v. and an antihistamine may help to alleviate shock. In the event of severe shock, support with intravenous adrenalin 1:10 000 in small incremental doses may be required. Further compatible transfusions may be required in severely affected patients. If acute renal failure occurs, this is managed in the usual way, if necessary with dialysis until recovery occurs.

MANAGEMENT OF PATIENTS WITH INFECTED BLOOD

Fortunately these reactions are rare. Treatment includes measures to combat shock. Antibiotic therapy, as appropriate, should be commenced as soon as the diagnosis is made and before culture results are known.

Other transfusion reactions

1 *Reactions due to white cell antibodies.* HLA antibodies (see below) are usually the result of sensitisation by pregnancy or a previous transfusion. They produce rigors, pyrexia and, in severe cases, pulmonary infiltrates. They may be minimised by giving leucocyte-depleted (e.g. filtered) packed cells.

2 *Allergic reactions* These are usually due to hypersensitivity to donor plasma proteins. The clinical features are urticaria, pyrexia and, in severe cases, dyspnoea, facial oedema and rigors. Immediate treatment is with antihistamines and hydrocortisone. Adrenalin is also useful. Washed red cells may be needed for further transfusions.

It is not possible to differentiate from the clinical symptoms the cause of many transfusion reactions. Laboratory tests are required and even these may fail to identify the mechanism for many allergic reactions.

3 *Post-transfusion circulatory overload.* The features include those of pulmonary oedema, fullness in the head, and dry cough. The management is that of cardiac failure. These reactions are prevented by a slow transfusion of packed red cells or of the blood component required, accompanied by diuretic therapy.

4 *Post-transfusion hepatitis.* This may be due to any of the hepatitis viruses, i.e. types A, B, non-A, non-B, and occasionally CMV and EB viruses have been implicated. Post-transfusion hepatitis is seen less frequently now because of routine HB_sAg testing of all blood donations.

5 *Acquired immune deficiency syndrome (AIDS).* This is a recently recognised disease most common in homosexual males in parts of North America. There is deficiency of helper T-lymphocytes with reversal of the normal suppressor:helper ratio $(T_8:T_4)$ in peripheral blood. Hypergammaglobulinaemia also occurs but the patient suffers recurrent severe infection, often with *Pneumocystis carinii*, herpes simplex, herpes zoster or other viruses or fungi. Kaposi's sarcoma is found with a high frequency. The disease appears to be rarely transmitted by blood transfusion and has been described in haemophilic patients receiving factor VIII concentrates. In its severe forms, the disease is usually fatal. The cause is now known to be infection with a chronic retrovirus, HTLV-III, which infects and destroys T_4 lymphocytes.

6 *Other infections.* Cytomegalovirus, infectious mononucleosis, toxoplasmosis, malaria and syphilis may all be transmitted by blood transfusion.

7 *Post-transfusional iron overload.* Repeated red cell transfusions over many years, in the absence of blood loss, cause deposition of iron in the reticulo-endothelial tissue at the rate of 200–250 mg per unit (450 ml) of whole blood. After 100 units in adults, and lesser amounts in children, the liver, myocardium and endocrine glands are damaged (see Chapter 2). This is a major problem in thalassaemia major (see Chapter 4) and other severe chronic refractory anaemias.

BANK BLOOD AND BLOOD PRODUCTS FOR TRANSFUSION

Donor blood is taken by an aseptic technique into plastic bags containing an appropriate amount of anticoagulant—usually citrate-phosphate-dextrose (CPD). The citrate anticoagulates the blood by combining with the blood calcium. Before issue the following tests are carried out: ABO and rhesus blood groups and antibody screen, serological tests to exclude syphilis and HB_sAg to exclude hepatitis B.

Blood is stored at 4–6°C and may be kept for 21–28 days. Many blood transfusion centres now use a red cell preservative fluid containing adenine-CPD which increases red cell storage to 28–35 days. After the first 48 hours there is a slow progressive K^+ loss from the red cells into the plasma. In cases where infusion of K^+ could be dangerous, fresh blood should be used, e.g. for exchange transfusion in haemolytic disease of the newborn. During red cell storage there is a fall in 2,3 diphosphoglycerate (2,3 DPG) and levels of this glycolytic pathway metabolite are significantly reduced or negligible after 28 days. Following transfusion, 2,3 DPG levels return to normal within 24 hours. The limiting factor in determining blood bank storage of red cells is the ability of the cells to circulate normally following transfusion. As the storage time increases, some red cells become spherical due to changes in energy metabolism. This is associated with an increase in red cell rigidity and after a period the cell injury becomes irreversible. If red cells are transfused at the time of maximum storage, up to 20–30% of the red cells may be destroyed within 24 hours, the remainder showing a survival close to normal.

Blood may be given whole or separated into its components. It is preferable to infuse only the necessary component, e.g. packed red cells for chronically anaemic patients.

Whole blood

This is usually reserved for treating acute blood loss, e.g. traumatic or surgical blood loss, severe gastrointestinal or uterine haemorrhage. In many small transfusions following acute blood loss (e.g. up to 2 units in adults) the use of packed cells plus electrolytes is often recommended rather than whole blood, in order to conserve plasma for other clinical uses.

Packed red cells

These are the treatment of choice in chronically anaemic patients who require transfusion. In older subjects, a diuretic is often given simultaneously and the infusion should be sufficiently slow to avoid circulatory overload. In the majority of patients with deficiency anaemias, iron, folate or B_{12} as appropriate is sufficient therapy and red cell transfusions are seldom required. In chronic anaemias which do not respond to haematinics, transfusion should be avoided unless the patient is at risk from or incapacitated by the anaemia. The haemoglobin level alone is not a good guide to transfusion need in view of the wide variation in cardiovascular adaptation and shift in O_2-dissociation curve between different individuals and different types of anaemia. Once regular transfusions have begun, iron chelation therapy with desferrioxamine should also be considered in an attempt to avoid iron overload.

Granulocyte concentrates

These are prepared on blood cell separators from normal healthy donors or from patients with chronic granulocytic leukaemia. Their use is restricted to patients with severe neutropenia ($< 0.5 \times 10^9/l$) who are not responding to antibiotic therapy (see p. 135). Localised infections respond best.

Platelet concentrates

These are harvested by cell separators or from several (usually six) donor units of blood. These concentrates are indicated in severely thrombocytopenic patients with established haemorrhage or prophylactically during intensive myelotoxic chemotherapy, as in acute leukaemia. Their most important use is therefore in the support of patients with severe aplastic anaemia or acute leukaemia. Occasionally they are required to provide temporary support in severe immune thrombocytopenia or in patients with severe acute disseminated intravascular coagulation, but their survival in these situations will be similar to that of the patient's own platelets, i.e. reduced to hours rather than days. ABO and Rh-compatible platelets are usually used but HLA-identical platelets are needed for patients with HLA antibodies.

Human plasma preparations

Plasma is a useful volume expander. The risk of hepatitis has been reduced in recent years due to the introduction of more sensitive tests for hepatitis B antigen. All frozen and dried plasma is usually prepared from single donor units.

FRESH FROZEN PLASMA. Rapidly frozen plasma separated from fresh blood is stored at $< -30°C$. Its main use is for the replacement of coagulation factors. If cryoprecipitate has been removed during its preparation it will be depleted in factors VIII and I and unsuitable for haemophilia treatment.

FRESH FREEZE-DRIED PLASMA. This is prepared from blood less than six hours old with levels of coagulation factors V and VIII approximately 50% of normal. It may be used as a plasma volume expander but is mainly used in treating suspected coagulation factor deficiency.

Stable plasma protein solution (SPPS) 5% or plasma protein fraction (PPF)

These solutions contain human albumin and globulin and are free from hepatitis risk. Their main use is in the treatment of shock.

They are recommended as the main general purpose plasma volume expanders, where a sustained osmotic effect is required prior to the administration of blood. They are also used for plasma replacement in patients undergoing plasmapheresis and sometimes for protein replacement in selected patients with hypoalbuminaemia.

Human albumin 25%

This expensive purified preparation is not recommended as a general plasma volume expander although its usefulness for this purpose is undoubted. It may be used in severe hypoalbuminaemia when it is necessary to use a product with minimal electrolyte content. Principal indications for its use are patients with the nephrotic syndrome or liver failure.

Cryoprecipitate

This is obtained by thawing fresh frozen plasma at $4°C$ and contains concentrated factor VIII and fibrinogen. It is stored at $< -30°C$ or, if lyophylised at $4-6°C$, and used as replacement therapy in haemophilia A and von Willebrand's disease.

Freeze-dried factor VIII concentrates

These are also used for treating haemophilia A. The small volume makes them ideal for children, surgical cases, patients at risk from circulatory overload and for those on home treatment.

Freeze-dried factor IX—prothrombin complex concentrates

A number of preparations are available which contain variable amounts of factors II, VII, IX and X. They are mainly used for treating factor IX deficiency (Christmas disease) but are also used occasionally in patients with liver disease or in life-threatening haemorrhage following overdose with oral anticoagulants.

Fibrinogen

This freeze-dried preparation is mainly prepared from time-expired plasma. It is used for treating fibrinogen deficiency, e.g. that associated with DIC following an obstetric emergency.

Immunoglobulin

Pooled immunoglobulin is a valuable source of antibodies against common viruses. It is used in hypogammaglobulinaemia for protection against viral and bacterial disease.

This may be obtained from donors with high titres of antibody, e.g. anti-rhesus D, anti-hepatitis B, anti-herpes zoster, anti-tetanus, anti-diphtheria.

ACUTE BLOOD LOSS

This is the commonest indication for whole blood transfusion. As mentioned on p. 17, until 3–4 hours after a single episode of blood loss, the Hb and PCV remain normal, since there is initial vasoconstriction with a reduction in total blood volume. After 3–4 hours, however, the plasma volume begins to expand and the Hb and PCV fall and there is a rise in neutrophils and platelets. The reticulocyte response begins on the 2nd or 3rd day and reaches a maximum of 10–15%, lasting 8–10 days. The haemoglobin begins to rise by about the 7th day but, if iron stores have become depleted, the haemoglobin may not rise subsequently to normal. Clinical assessment is needed to gauge whether blood transfusion is needed, but this is usually unnecessary with losses of 500 ml or less unless haemorrhage is continuing. Blood transfusion is not without risks and should not be undertaken lightly.

HAEMOLYTIC DISEASE OF THE NEWBORN

Haemolytic disease of the newborn (HDN) is the result of passage of IgG antibodies from the maternal circulation across the placenta into the circulation of the foetus where they react with and damage foetal red cells.

Before 1967 and the introduction of prophylactic use of IgG, anti-D rhesus HDN was responsible for about 800 stillbirths and neonatal deaths each year in the U.K. Anti-D was responsible for 94% of rhesus HDN; other cases were usually due to anti-c and ante-E, with a wide range of antibodies found in occasional cases (for examples see Table 14.1). The incidence of rhesus HDN is now dramatically lower and the proportion of cases due to anti-c and anti-E has increased substantially.

The most frequent causes of HDN are now immune antibodies of the ABO blood group system—most commonly anti-A produced by a group O mother against a group A foetus. However, this form of HDN is usually mild. More severely affected infants are treated with exchange transfusion and phototherapy described below. Antenatal tests on maternal blood are unreliable in predicting the severity of HDN but do indicate which women need close monitoring.

Occasional cases of HDN are caused by antibodies of other blood group systems, e.g. anti-Kell.

PATHOGENESIS OF RHESUS-D HDN

A Rh-D negative (Rh d/d or rr) woman has a pregnancy with a rhesus-D positive foetus. Rh-D positive foetal red cells cross into the maternal circulation (usually at parturition) and sensitise the mother to form anti-D. Sensitisation is more likely if the mother and foetus are ABO compatible. The mother could also be sensitised by a previous miscarriage, amniocentesis or blood transfusion.

Anti-D crosses the placenta to the foetus during the next pregnancy with a rhesus-D-positive foetus, coats the foetal red cells with antibody and results in destruction of these cells, causing anaemia and jaundice. If the father is heterozygous for D antigen (D/d) there is a 50% probability that the foetus will be D positive.

CLINICAL FEATURES

(i) *Severe disease:* intrauterine death from hydrops foetalis.
(ii) *Moderate disease:* the baby is born with severe anaemia and jaundice and may show pallor, tachycardia, oedema and hepato-splenomegaly. When the unconjugated bilirubin level exceeds 250 mmol/l bile pigment deposition in the basal ganglia may lead to kernicterus — central nervous system damage with generalised spasticity and possible subsequent mental deficiency, deafness and epilepsy. This problem becomes acute after birth as maternal clearance of foetal bilirubin ceases and conjugation of bilirubin by the neonatal liver has to be induced to reach full activity.
(iii) *Mild disease:* mild anaemia with or without jaundice.

LABORATORY FINDINGS AT BIRTH

(i) *Cord blood.* Variable anaemia (haemoglobin < 18/dl) with a high reticulocyte count; the baby is Rh-D positive, the direct Coombs' test is positive and the serum bilirubin raised.
(ii) *The mother* is Rh-D negative with a high plasma titre of anti-D.

TREATMENT

Exchange transfusion may be necessary; the indications for this include:
Clinical features: obvious pallor, jaundice and signs of heart failure.
Laboratory findings: Hb < 14.0 g/dl with a positive direct Coombs' test; a cord serum bilirubin > 60 mmol/l or infant serum bilirubin greater than 300 mmol/l (18.0 mg/100 ml) or bilirubin level rising

rapidly and Coombs' test positive. Premature babies are more liable to kernicterus and should be exchange transfused at lower bilirubin levels (e.g. > 200 mmol/l).

In infants with moderate disease, more than one exchange transfusion may be required. Exchange transfusions performed soon after birth are used to replace the infant's red cells and reduce the rate of bilirubin rise. Subsequent exchange transfusions may be required to remove unconjugated bilirubin. The procedure of removing and replacing one equivalent blood volume will remove 60% of the pre-existing constituents in the blood. The blood for the exchange transfusion should be fresh Rh-D negative and ABO compatible with the baby and with the mother's serum by cross-match. Normally, 500 ml is sufficient for each exchange. Phototherapy (exposure of the infant to bright light of appropriate wavelength) has been used to photo-degrade the bilirubin to permit urinary excretion, thus reducing the likelihood of kernicterus.

MANAGEMENT OF PREGNANT WOMEN

1 At the time of booking all pregnant women should have their ABO and rhesus group determined and serum screened for antibodies. Rh-D negative women should have serum re-checked for antibodies in each trimester (e.g. at initial presentation, 24 weeks and 36 weeks). In women with antibody, the identity of the antibody should be checked and the specificity and titre re-checked at regular intervals (e.g. 4-weekly, and more often in late pregnancy or if antibody levels are rising or high).

2 The severity of the haemolytic disease can be assessed by spectroscopic estimation of bile pigment derivatives in the amniotic fluid obtained by amniocentesis. If this shows severe haemolysis the foetus can be kept alive by intrauterine transfusion of fresh Rh-D negative blood after 24 weeks and by premature delivery after 35 weeks.

3 Suitable fresh blood should be available at the time of induction in preparation for exchange transfusion.

4 At birth the babies of Rh-D negative women who do not have antibodies must have their cord blood grouped for ABO and rhesus. If the baby's blood is Rh-D negative the mother will require no further treatment.

5 *Prevention of Rh immunization.* Passively administered IgG anti-D suppresses primary immunisation in Rh-D negative women. Anti-D is now given to every Rh-D negative woman giving birth to an Rh-D positive child providing the woman has not been previously sensitised. The routine dose is 100 μg i.m. within 72 hours of delivery.

A Kleihauer test may be performed to estimate the severity of the foeto-maternal bleed. This uses differential staining to estimate the number of foetal cells in the maternal circulation (Fig. 14.2). The chance of developing antibodies is related to the number of foetal cells found. The dose of anti-D is increased if the Kleihauer test shows greater than 4 ml transplacental haemorrhage. To

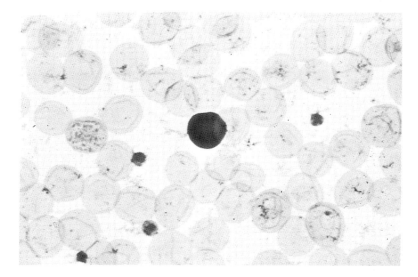

Fig. 14.2 Kleihauer test for foetal red cells. A deeply eosin-staining cell containing foetal haemoglobin is seen at the centre. Haemoglobin has been eluted from the other red cells by incubation at acid pH and these appear as colourless ghosts.

women having an abortion at under 12 weeks of pregnancy, 50 µg anti-D is given and, in those after 12 weeks, the usual dose of 100 µg is given. Similar treatment should also be given in threatened abortion and in the case of amniocentesis performed on Rh-D negative women. Some national variation exists in the size of doses employed, and depends partly on the availability of therapeutic anti-D.

THE HUMAN LEUCOCYTE ANTIGEN (HLA) SYSTEM

The short arm of chromosome 6 contains a cluster of genes known as the major histocompatibility complex or the HLA region (see Fig. 14.3). Amongst the genes in this region are those that determine the structure of the HLA antigens, which are present on the membrane surface of most nucleated cells, and which are known to provoke severe reactions when tissues or organs are exchanged between genetically non-identical people. It is now known that this region codes not only for the HLA antigens, but also for several components of the complement cascade, and a number of so-called immune response genes which (at least in mice) appear to determine the strength of humoral and cellular immune responses to soluble antigens. The gene cluster is adjacent to the loci occupied by the genes for several enzymes and this information has been used in gene mapping studies.

There are at least four separate allelic series of HLA antigens (Fig. 14.3). HLA-A and HLA-B phenotypes are determined with typing sera obtained from subjects sensitised by previous transfusion or pregnancy. The weaker HLA-C system may also be deter-

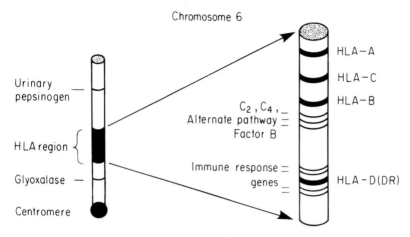

Fig. 14.3 The human leucocyte antigen (HLA) gene complex. HLA-A, -B and -C antigens are termed Class 1 and HLA-D antigens (now divided into DP, DQ and DR) are termed Class 2.

mined by serological methods. The HLA-A, -B and -C antigens are present on the surface membranes of all nucleated cells; they are also present on platelets and may sometimes be present on red cells. HLA-A, -B and -C typing is usually carried out on peripheral blood lymphocytes. Originally, antigens at the major lymphocyte activating locus, HLA-D, were identified by looking for non-reactivity in a mixed lymphocyte culture (MLC) reaction (a lymphocyte proliferation assay) against rare homozygous D locus cells. The restricted availability of these cells prevented the use of this MLC test for routine HLA-D typing. More recently it was discovered that the sera of multiparous women and patients who had received multiple transfusions contained antibodies which appeared to recognise eight of the eleven known HLA-D antigens. Until these antigens defined by serology have been proven biochemically to be the same as those defined by the MLC typing method, it has been decided to refer to them as HLA-DR (D related) antigens. The HLA-DR antigens are restricted in tissue distribution to B-lymphocytes, macrophages and some endothelial cells. HLA-DR typing is carried out usually on peripheral blood or splenic lymphocyte populations from which the T-lymphocytes have been removed.

The inheritance of the four loci (HLA-A, -B, -C and -DR) is closely linked; one set of loci is inherited from each parent so that there is a 1 in 4 chance of two siblings having identical HLA antigens (Fig 14.4). HLA is the most polymorphic system of genes yet discovered in man. Currently there are known to be 17 HLA-A alleles, more than 30 HLA-B alleles, 6 HLA-C alleles, 11 HLA-D alleles and 8 HLA-DR alleles, together with a number of less well defined alleles.

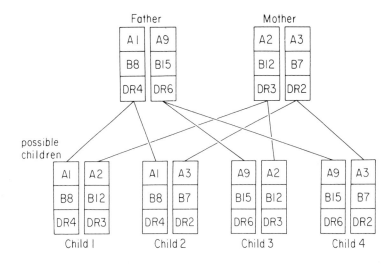

Fig. 14.4 An example of possible pattern of inheritance of the A, B and DR series alleles of the HLA complex.

HLA and transplantation

The main practical application of HLA typing has been in the selection of donor–recipient pairs for renal transplantation and more recently for bone marrow transplantation. Although immunological rejection always occurs unless donor and recipient are identical twins, the severity of rejection is known to be influenced by the degree of compatibility between the tissue of the donor and the recipient. When renal grafts are exchanged between HLA-identical siblings, a minimal degree of rejection occurs which may be controlled by immunosuppressive drugs and the success rate is high. The rejection response is directed against other weaker antigenic differences between the transplanted organ and the host. However, most renal grafts are from unrelated cadaver donors and perfect HLA matches are almost impossible. However, grafts well matched for the HLA-A, HLA-B, and HLA-DR antigens survive

significantly better than poorly matched grafts. The selection procedure for renal transplantation is guided by the following rules:
1. The donor should be ABO compatible,
2. The donor and recipient should be as closely HLA matched as possible,
3. There should be a negative lymphocytoxicity cross-match between the recipient's serum and the donor's lymphocytes (i.e. HLA-A, -B, -C and -DR cross-match).

The requirements for successful bone marrow transplantation are more rigid, for added to the problems of acute graft rejection are those of graft-versus-host disease. Even when the marrow donor is an HLA-identical sibling and there is no reactivity in the MLC test, graft-versus-host disease may still occur. This may be due to other histocompatibility systems not linked to HLA. Much poorer results with unrelated donors, however well matched, must reflect genetic differences which are inaccessible to present typing techniques.

HLA and blood transfusion

Since the HLA-A, -B and -C antigens are carried by leucocytes and platelets, each transfusion of whole blood, platelet or leucocyte concentrate carries the risk of immunising the patient to these antigens; immunisation may also follow pregnancy. Immunisation against HLA antigens may cause febrile, non-haemolytic transfusion reactions (see p. 247). These may be minimised by removing with filters most of the white cells and platelets from the red cells prior to transfusion. Immunisation may also result in failure of patients to respond to transfusion of leucocyte and platelet concentrates with the expected rise in cell counts. Once immunisation has

Table 14.6 HLA and disease associations.

Disease	HLA-antigen	Relative risk
Ankylosing spondylitis	B27	91
Coeliac disease	DR3	73
Reiter's disease	B27	36
Subacute thyroiditis	Bw35	17
Dermatitis herpetiformis	DR3	14
Idiopathic haemochromatosis	A3	9
Addison's disease	DR3	9
Behçet's disease	B5	7
Psoriasis	Cw6	6
Multiple sclerosis	DR2	4
Rheumatoid arthritis	DR4	4
Juvenile diabetes	DR3,4	3
Chronic active hepatitis	B8	3

occurred, concentrates should be prepared from HLA-identical family members using cell separators.

HLA and disease

Since the initial report in 1973 that 96% of patients suffering from ankylosing spondolytis carry the HLA-B27 antigen, more than 100 diseases have been shown to have an association with HLA. Some of the most important associations are shown in Table 14.6. There are as yet no proven explanations for these associations, although they clearly relate to the central role of the HLA gene complex and immunological responsiveness, and imply that HLA type is relevant to susceptibility or resistance to specific diseases.

SELECTED BIBLIOGRAPHY

British Medical Bulletin (1978) *The HLA,System*, vol. 34.
Clinics in Haematology (1976) vol. 5.1, *Blood Transfusion and Blood Products*. Ed. J.D. Cash. W.B. Saunders, Philadelphia.
Dausset J. & Svejgaard (1977) *HLA and Disease*. Munksgaard, Copenhagen.
Festenstein H. & Dèmant P. (1978) *HLA and H-2. Basic Immunogenetics, Biology and Clinical Relevance*. Edward Arnold, London.
Miller W.V. (1977) The human histocompatibility complex: A review for the hematologist. In *Progress in Haematology*, vol. X, p. 173. Grune and Stratton, New York.
Mollison P.L. (1982) *Blood Transfusion in Clinical Medicine*, 7th edition. Blackwell Scientific Publications, Oxford.
Race R.R. & Sanger R. (1975) *Blood Groups in Man*, 6th edition. Blackwell Scientific Publications, Oxford.
Wallace J. (1977) *Blood Transfusion for Clinicians*. Churchill Livingstone, Edinburgh.
Worlledge S. (1981) Blood Group Serology, Antigens in Human Blood, Practical Blood Transfusion. In *Postgraduate Haematology*, eds. A.V. Hoffbrand & S.M. Lewis, pp. 269-380. Heinemann Medical, London.
Major textbooks of haematology (see Chapter 1).

Index